PSYCHIC

EMPATH

Psychic Development Survival Guide for Highly Sensitive People! Practicing Mindfulness, Mental Health Essential Meditations and Affirmations to Reduce Stress and Find Your Sense of Self

BY

Jack Gross

TABLE OF CONTENTS

COPYRIGHTS

This book

"PSYCHIC EMPATH: Psychic Development Survival Guide for Highly Sensitive People. Practicing Mindfulness, Mental Health Essential Meditations and Affirmations to Reduce Stress and Find Your Sense of Self

Written by Jack Gross

This Document aims to provide precise and reliable details on this subject and the problem under discussion.

The product has marketed on the assumption that no officially approved bookkeeping or publishing house provides other available funds.

Where a legal or qualified guide is required, a person must have the right to participate in the field.

A statement of principle, which is a subcommittee of the American Bar Association, a committee of publishers and Associations and approved. A copy, reproduction, or distribution of parts of this text, in electronic or written form, is not permitted.

The recording of this Document is strictly prohibited, and retention of this text is only with the written permission of the publisher and all Liberties authorized.

The information provided here is correct and reliable, as any lack of attention or other means resulting from the misuse or use of the procedures, procedures, or instructions contained therein is the total, and absolute obligation of the user addressed.

The author is not obliged, directly or indirectly, to assume civil or civil liability for any restoration, damage, or loss resulting from the data collected here. The respective authors retain all copyrights not kept by the publisher.

The information contained herein is solely and universally available for information purposes. The data is presented without a warranty or promise of any kind.

The trademarks used are without approval, and the patent is issued without the trademark owner's permission or protection.

The logos and labels here are the possessions of the owners themselves and are not associated with this text.

CHAPTER 1: INTRODUCTION TO PSYCHIC EMPATH

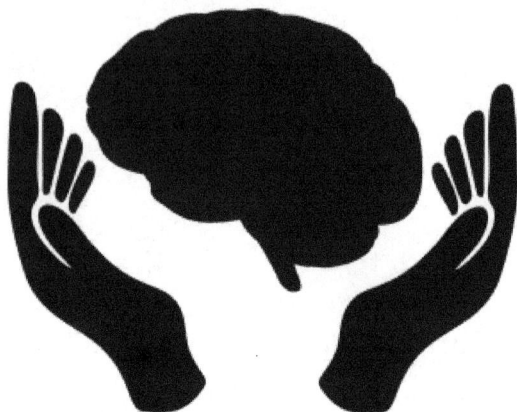

I have been in Native Medicine for 14 years at USC and UCLA, and I am also an empathizer. In my health care for over 20 years, I've been specializing in treating susceptible people like me. Humans have different sensitivities, but empathy is an emotional sponge that absorbs both the stress and joy of the world. We all feel extreme; there is little protection between others and us. As a result, we are often overwhelmed by overstimulation, which tends to lead to fatigue and sensory overload. I'm so passionate about this topic both professionally and personally because I've had to develop specific strategies to manage the challenges of being an empath myself. These allow me to protect my sensitivities so I can maximize their benefits — and there are so many! I want to share with you how to become a balanced, empowered, and happy empath. To thrive, you must learn ways to avoid taking on the energy, symptoms, and stress of others. I also want to educate your loved ones and peers — family, coworkers, bosses, parents, and romantic partners — on how best to support and communicate with you. In this book, I will show you how to accomplish these goals.

I provide the Campus Survival Guide as a resource for the relevant sensitive souls to find understanding and acceptance in a world often harsh, heartless, and painful. In it, we challenge the status quo and create new normality to show sensitivity anywhere in the spectrum. There is nothing "wrong" about being sensitive. You are trying to understand what is "right" for you. In this book, the Empaths essential tools, and the Empaths workshops, I would like to find a tribe and create a community of support that is genuine and shining. I want to support the movement of people who respect their sensibility. Welcome to the circle of love! My message to you is one of hope and acceptance. We encourage you to accept the gifts and do your best to empathize with them.

Empath

The sympathetic nerve has a very reactive nervous system. Filters to block stimulation are not the same as others. As a result, we absorb both joyous and stressful energies around us in our bodies. We are so sensitive that it's like having fifty fingers instead of five. We are super responders. Studies show varying degrees of susceptibility, but high sensitivity affects approximately 20% of the population. As children and adults, we are ashamed of our sensitivity rather than our support. We can experience chronic fatigue, which often feels overwhelming, so we want to withdraw from the world. But at this point in our life, I shouldn't give up on being empathetic to anything. It makes us feel the secret of the universe and lets us know the passion beyond our dreams. But our empathy didn't always seem so incredible to us.

Common Types of Empathy

Physical empathies are especially prone to the physical symptoms of others and tend to absorb them into your body. The well-being of a person can also energize them. Emotional empathy. They mainly absorb the emotions of others and can be a sponge of happy and sad feelings. Experience incredible perceptions of intuition, telepathy, dream messages, flora and fauna communication, contact with others. The different types and their functions are listed below. Today, telepathic empathy receives intuitive information about others.

Precognitive empathy has a warning about the future while waking up and dreaming. Dream sympathizers are enthusiastic dreamers who can receive intuitive information from dreams to help others and lead them into their lives. Plant empathy can sense plant needs and connect with the essence of plants. Earth's path adapts to changes in the Earth, solar system, and weather. Animal sympathizers can adapt to and communicate with animals.

Sympathetic people have a distinct, beautiful, and subtle sense. These can be one or more of the above types. The next chapters will also discuss specific types of physical and emotional empathy, including the food empathy (matching the energy of the food) and relationship and sexual compassion (matching the mood of partners and friends), sensuality, physical health). If you learn to identify your unique talents, you will find that they not only enrich your life but can also be helpful for the benefit of others.

How to Tell You Are One?

Do you have a direct connection with people, places, or animals? Do you trust people you know little about, with greater confidence?

Such a painful experience can be due to empathy. You may be a psychological companion if you immediately see the personality of the person you just met or have a similar experience. To empathize is to understand and share the emotions of others as if they were in the same position. Empathy is someone susceptible to the energy around him and the feelings of people and animals. It includes spiritual footprints and the mental strength of the place. Empathians have a unique ability with an evident emotion called fluoroscopy. Fluoroscopy is the ability to feel the emotions present in the world when interacting with people, places, and animals. Sympathizers are firmly in tune with the energy around them. It means that they are sensitive to the strength of others, plants, places, and animals.

Types of Psychic Empaths

Not all sympathizers have the same skills. Some sympathizers can feel the emotions inside of fellow humans, while others can perceive subtle changes in energy levels around them. However, all empathizers, in stock, can handle these energy levels and adapt to subtle changes that other non-sympathizers often do not see or notice. The type of empathy you have determines what kind of emotional heart you have. Types of understanding and their skills are as explained below:

Emotional Empath

This type of empathy has some of the most common types of kindness. Emotional understanding allows you to absorb the sensitive emotions of fellow humans and experience them for yourself.

This feature can help others. It makes empathy a great listener because you can say that you know where somebody came from, even if it's not what they've experienced. However, this feature can quickly become exhausted, for example, when you are near a person who is experiencing great sadness. The most critical thing to remember is to distinguish your feelings from the feelings of others around you and protect yourself from being overly influenced by beliefs that do not belong to you. Geographical empathy is also called environmental understanding. You may have this ability if you feel happy or uncomfortable in a situation or environment for no apparent reason. There may also be deep connections to specific locations and places of power such as churches and grove.

Physical/Medical Empathy

You can become a physical or medical empathy if you intuitively know the energy other people are feeling—many people with this ability, whether traditional or alternative careers, seek healing to help others. If you think you are a physical companion, you need to be aware of how these skills affect your body. If you feel the energy of others in yourself, you may have a severe health problem or an existing problem.

Plant Empathy

A plant's insight is someone who instinctively knows what a plant need. You can also sit on a specific tree and meditate to deepen your bond and deepen your understanding.

The Sympathy of animals

Strong relationships with animals indicate that you are an animal sympathizer. Animal empathy is devoted to the care of animals, and often they have a better understanding of what they need and want. Some people can even communicate with animals telepathically.

Intuitive / Claircognizant Empath

Intuitive empathy can gather a lot of information from someone by merely being in front of them and sometimes looking at them. For example, you can feel the meaning and intent behind what you learned, so you can quickly see when someone is trying to lie to you and when. If you scan the energy of fellow humans, you will feel the need to surround yourself with others with powers that match your life.

CHAPTER 2: HIGHLY SENSITIVE PEOPLE AND PSYCHIC DEVELOPMENT

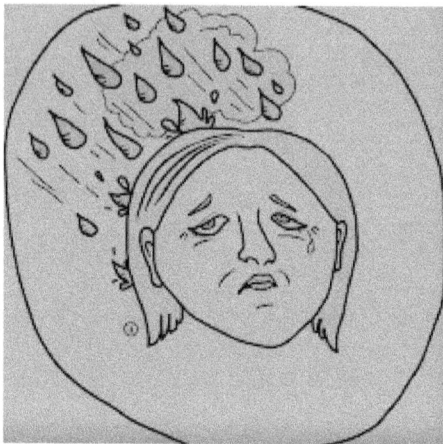

In the 1990s, psychologist Elaine Aron discovered a new group of people and called them susceptible people (Aron, 1996). According to Soons, Brouwers, and Tomic (2010), "sensitivity refers to the ability to perceive neutral or emotionally weak stimuli from the environment, one's body, or one's perception." As an example, Soons et al. (2010) showed that Highly sensitive people (HSPs) might notice subtle emotional changes in tone, sound, and pitch outside the non-HSP range. Other physical reactions affecting HSPs include increased sensitivity to light, hunger, temperature, caffeine, and drugs (Aron & Aron, 1997; Vaughan, 2016). Besides, in 2015, Markowitz found that most HSPs felt the need to heal the physical and emotional pain of others for insightful intuition and compassion. Markowitz added that the responsibility for treating others negatively impacts HSP's immune system and energy fields. As a result, duty brought HSP angry, embarrassed, and guilty. Vaughan added that HSPs often felt they were out of sync with society.

Vaughn found that HSP's gifts included increased creativity and artistic ability, intuition, the potential for empathy and care, and a high need for spiritual connections. Aron developed a highly sensitive self-test to identify and measure the typical characteristics of highly sensitive people. The self-test included questions about whether a person was a little scared, whether they were affected by the mood of others, and whether teachers and parents found him shy or sensitive. Highly sensitive people (HSPs) make up 15-20% of the population and can read, resonate, and understand the emotional state of others. Aron suggested that people may consider HSPs to be shy, weak, withdrawn, or unreliable. In 2004, Zeff indicated that when HSPs experience subtle affective disorders and negative energies, they feel unprepared and resistant. If the HSP feels unprepared, it is challenging to consider an intuitive experience as a positive personality trait. In 2011, Bartz reported that

HSPs tend to see personality susceptibility as a disorder because they feel rejected by the majority of non-HSP populations. Similarly, Aron found that HSPs thought was separated from 75-80% of society. Aron discovered that unpredictable environmental stimuli such as screaming sirens, bright lights, and emotional energy affect people in a 21st-century community.

However, these stressors affected HSPs more than non-HSPs. In 2011, Chevalier and Sinatra identified the Autonomic Nervous System (ANS) as a cause of emotional hypersensitivity in the human body, suggesting that 21st-century stress increasingly affects ANS and physiological status in all humans. Aron indicated that the sensitive nature of the HSP nervous system led to an unintentionally enhanced absorption of stimulants that could disrupt the thinking process of HSPs. For example,

Zeff found that HSP felt more pain and might have investigated the cause of the problem. Due to the intuitive nature of HSP (Aron, 1996), HSP instinctively knew a potential friend or potential enemy. Zeff explained that HSPs are friendly, caring, understandable, and natural advisors, teachers, and healers. In addition to the caring nature of HSP, Zeff has discovered that HSP is enthusiastic and grateful for love, art, beauty, spirituality, and joy.

According to Bartz in 2011, most HSPs experience higher emotional stimuli and understand the need for a certain amount of rest, deep internal processing, and natural creativity. However, some consider the need for HSPs for internal processing to be introverted. According to Grimen and Diseth in 2016, and Aron state that HSPs are so stimulating that they process details simultaneously at the internal level. While

Adler, Freud, and Jung classified the differences between introverted and extroverted behavior.

Aron explained that HSPs have four primary functions. HSPs learn to recognize significant features and are thus more sensitive to defective components. Aron encouraged HSPs to recognize predominant features when they were exposed. The cheap function is to believe in the thoughts of others (even if it is not true). Another inferior quality is projecting inferiority and self-doubt to others. Aron thought that the inadequacy of HSP ended with self-love and patience.

At the spiritual level, people can call HSP empathetic. In 2015, Markowitz explained that empathy could intuitively observe others, raising awareness of subtle differences, and increasing compassion for others. The HSP recognizes subtleties that may go unnoticed, but most of the population may not be able to identify susceptible people because of the HSP.

Usually, we feel the pressure to hide their sensitivity. This increase in emotional vulnerability can reduce self-confidence and self-esteem. But in 2016, Sand stated that the personal exposure of HSPs increased compassion and empathy. Similarly, Aron found that HSP's recognition of others increased understanding and explanation of social justice. Sand said: "If we can connect to more vulnerable emotions, we can shift energy and create more space for the healing process."

Heredity and Nature

Compassionate personality can set up in over 100 species and an estimated 20%. Aron discovered that high sensitivity is an intrinsic property designed to survive (quoted from Acevedo et al., 2014). Aron saw that HSPs display sensory processing sensitivity (SPS) in response to social and environmental stimuli. Aron suggested that "SPS is increasingly associated with identifiable genes, behaviors, physiological responses, and patterns of brain activation."

Besides, SPS was a natural survival tactic for all species, animals to respond immediately to dangerous and evolving situations. If the species bring into being the same, and there was no difference in personality, they predicted that they could be extinct. The sensory processing sensitivities of HSPs include increased consciousness, increased responsiveness, and empathy due to increased activation in various brain regions. Terazawa, Moriguchi, Tochizawa, Umeda in 2014, discovered that HSP's nerve impulse (intuition) could perceive HSP's emotions of others through human facial expressions, and even mild anger and disgust.

Impact of Parents and Care

A limited study of sensitive personalities began in 1991 by Aron. In 1997, he found that the newly developed HSP scale was reliable and competent. Aron investigated susceptible children (HSCs) and discovered whether parental care affects HSK and whether they mature into highly vulnerable adults. Participants in Aron included HSCs living at home with mental illness or alcoholism. Aron found patterns that led to negative emotions, such as temperamental behavior. Negative affection was the term Aron used to describe the adverse effects of parents. Aron confirmed that children raised in a supportive, positive, and caring environment were more likely to have social interactions and non-HSP traits in adulthood.

According to Chunhui et al. in 2011, "Researchers have found that exposure to family environments and stressful life events enhances susceptibility." The hypothesis is that environmental effects cause personality changes. They tested a multi-step approach at the nervous system level, evaluated dopamine-related genes and environmental factors, and assessed how they contributed to HSP traits. Chunhui et al. personality depend on the dopaminergic response of the neuronal system, which gives an account to be genetically associated with personality and stress.

In 2011, they discovered that the HSP dopamine gene contributed to the unpredictability of HSP personality. Like Chunhui et al., A study by Aron in 2004 showed that genetic features of HSPs did not induce introversion, shyness, or suppression unless negative parental sentiment comprised in HSP childhood. Using the Parental Warmth and Acceptance Scale (PWAS), "An empathetic personality does not correlate with parental warmth but is significantly and positively associated with the number of stressful life events in middle school and college."

Environment and Chios

An empathetic personality is intuitively hypersensitive to the surroundings (Meindl, n.d.c). Due to the hypersensitivity of HSP, Meindl suggested that HSP is more susceptible to stress, depression, and other mental health problems. Meindl described physical symptoms such as fast heart rate, heavy chest sensations, and intense pressure. In 2015, Cooper explained that HSPs contributed to increased emotional internal sensitivity to psychological coordination and management difficulties. Cooper told that adjusting emotions is difficult for HSPs. Cooper figuratively compared the dynamic response of HSP with a thermometer that quickly reaches the boiling point. Cooper stressed that HSP's difficulty in coordinating emotions created stigma leading to terms such as madness, neurosis, bipolar disorder, and personality disorder.

In 1996, Aron believed that the insensitivity of others led to a common misunderstanding about the personality and emotional needs of HSPs. Deci and Ryan have found that society does not support HSP's psychological need for autonomy, connection, and attribution (quoted from Cooper, 2015). For example, HSPs may find it necessary to compensate for the lack of connectivity and the ability to function in a social environment. Aron described the need for the temporary interruption of HSP and withdrawal from society. For example, the HSP may need to create a brief and safe place to recover and balance energy. As Meindl pointed out, there are four areas of overstimulation that cause stress in HSPs.

Meindl's first type of hyperstimulation is chronic environmental hyperstimulation. Meindl reported that overstimulation is not offensive to anyone. A person may be unable to leave an intense and stimulating environment. Firefighters, for example, are in such a difficult situation that they cannot issue a burning house. Similarly, HSP mothers cannot leave their children because of their stubborn behavior. As a result, Meindl found that the inability to control overstimulation increases the risk of potential feelings of helplessness, numbness, and depression.

The second type of overstimulation is hypersensitivity. Hypersensitivity is an acute awareness of physiological responses and emotional energy in an individual's environment. For example, hypersensitive

HSPs are more sensitive to internal stimuli and thus more susceptible to anxiety and depression. The third type of HSP overstimulation involved an abundant inner life with the ability to process accurate intuition. The HSP could anticipate danger and avoid potential problems, as well as access to detailed insights and precise intuition. Meindl suggested that the psychological abilities of HSPs created overwhelming emotions that contribute to depression and anxiety.

The fourth type of hyperstimulation in Meindl is interpersonal hyperstimulation. For example, Meindl discovered that HSPs had improved the ability to process the unconscious and conscious feelings of others. For example, HSP unknowingly reflects the emotions of others and can lead to depression or illness when dealing with someone who has these symptoms. Features of compassionate personality Aron (2004) argued that HSPs could be described as shy by their sizeable internal structure, attention to detail, and timely cognitive processing. Cooper has concluded that most of humanity is insensitive and extroverted. Therefore, surviving in this environment can be a daunting task for HSPs. Howes (2016) believed that when HSP interpersonal and hyperstimulation occurred, HSPs needed additional time to respond, reflect their thoughts, and clarify. Reported by Tarc (2013): "I use the term "inner life" to describe the "boundary space between the physical and social worlds between human unconsciousness and fanciful and expressible thoughts. For example, HSPs live in this interior space, are fully present, and can access and express a variety of potential emotions. Cooper (2014) also believed that HSPs have the gift of confronting them because they unintentionally feel the energy and feelings of others. Hinter Berger, Zlabinger, and Blaser (2014) called the mentalization of this type of unintended processing. Mentalization is also the ability to process external information through an internal focus.

To respond honestly to social pressures, HSPs try to feel comfortable when they hide their sensibilities from others. In 2015, Cooper further discovered that rejection pervades all entities in the HSP Life Experience. The emotions of rejection caused painful and complex emotions that took years to overcome. The result is an imbalance in the spirit of HSP. The cognitive inequality continued until the HSP accepted its sensitivity.

Jung's theory argued that an introverted personality type integration process (like HSP's emotional susceptibility) could take a lifetime to adapt to an extroverted (non-HSP) society. The HSP unknowingly absorbed the emotions of others, so the HSP felt responsible for the burden of others. As a result, HSPs developed low self-esteem due to the absorption of negative energy. As a result, in 2016, Sand found that most HSPs had no social connection.

Highly Sensitive Personalities and Individual Psychology

Adler's psychology positioned on the concept of social concern (Edgar, 1975). Social anxiety refers to behavior and attitudes within a community of work and personal relationships. Adler promoted collective empathy and sincere social interest. He further explained insight as to the ability to walk in the position of others and came to understand how their behavior affected others in society. Adler's therapeutic tools include collective empathy that contributes to the development of life challenges, attracts sincere social interest, reveals childhood memory, and identifies false beliefs. His treatment gives people a positive social sentiment, which enables them to remember themselves and accept social acceptance around the world. He added that social empathy promotes a sense of belonging, responsibility, and collaboration for the well-being of all community members (quoted by Ansbacher in 1956). Community success involved understanding and contributing to the three tasks of life: work, love, and social issues (Carlson, Watts & Maniacci, 2006). Similarly, Aron said there is a need to understand how HSPs respond in professional, personal, and social relationships. However, the concept of social concern and the resolution of municipal issues can be difficult for susceptible people.

A person is very sensitive to social interests. He believed that social interaction involves individual behavior in the context of peers, personal relationships, culture, and community. Adler explained that it's optimistic confidence in yourself and a real concern for the well-being and happiness of others. Mosak and Maniacci in 1999, state that social interest includes responsible behavior towards others, empathic attachment, and individual attitudes towards others.

Aron argued that today's cultural and social frameworks are not always safe places for HSPs (quoted from Satiroglu, 2008). In other words, HSPs are often excluded and misunderstood by peer groups. After interviewing HSP, Satiroglu (2008) reported that HSP pretended to wear a mask so that his peers would accept it. For example, this stone face mask had no emotion. Zeff assumed that HSP men should avoid sensitive behavior. As mentioned earlier, Zeff found that HSPs have an increased ability to negatively overstimulate the mood and tone of others, especially in intimate relationships. For example, Aron found that HSP fell in love and was more deeply hurt when a connection failed. Aron suggested that when HSP was in love, the couple had to engage in social activities rather than isolate themselves due to this sensitive nature. Also, Aron felt that HSP couples should not be overly responsive to each other's actions and irritability while attending a reception. Cooper (2015) said HSPs felt unavoidable and tired while absorbing the energy of others, so they felt the need to withdraw from large gatherings. Cooper also states that "HSP is a very minor and is often outside the realm of what is considered" normal "behavior. Cooper argued that everyone must feel gratitude, support, and love to experience a sense of belonging. Similarly, Zeff (2004) concluded that if HSPs were vulnerable to an unhealthy and unacceptable environment, they could not maintain the joyful feelings, and the relationship would deteriorate.

Aslinia, Rasheed, and Simpson in 2011 said Adler claimed that individuals were creative, unified, and social. Adler said that an ideal society allows individuals to feel accepted and positively contribute to the community. Adler (1933/2005) believed that everyone deserves a sense of belonging. As an example, He explained that individuals should not browbeat by the ideal image of society (or what other people think is normal). Adler also emphasized that collaboration and acceptance by others creates a balance of individual and community needs. Moreover, both individuals and communities thrive on social contributions.

Adler found that most people in society had an innate desire to pursue meaning (cited by Abramson, 2015). Moreover, He believed that all people overcome obstacles by changing their perspectives, thoughts, and feelings. According to Aslinia et al., it encouraged Adler to shift from weak emotions (perceived to be negative) to the right, capable emotions (perceived to be positive). As a result, neurosis, depression, anxiety, and inferiority live in useless aspects of life (inferior emotions). Remarkably low feelings keep going by misunderstandings of yourself, others, and the world (Adler, 1933/2005). Overholser (2010) said Adler believes that avoiding social interactions is a natural consequence of neurosis.

Inferiority Complex

Adler believed that neither heredity nor the environment had an impact on lifestyle development (Overholser, cited 2010). Also, Adler argued that interpreting life experiences and attitudes toward the world contributed to lifestyle development. Adler also believed that the individual's understanding of his or her strengths and weaknesses would increase the likelihood of achieving and accomplishing the goals of life. Adler explained that inferior sentiment was a subjective and overall assessment of the deficit (Carlson et al., 2006). According to Adler (1933/2005), the feeling of inferiority correlates with a person's sense of inadequacy. Carlson (2006) added that defense mechanisms, such as the immune system, are used to overcompensate weak emotions. Moreover, low feelings affect the achievement of life goals. Through social training, Adler learns to reveal, confront, and redesign the personal view of himself and others (Adler, quoted in 2005).

Moreover, Adler considered social training to be the best way to enable the positive movements needed to achieve life goals. Cooper (2015) found that 48% of HSPs feel different in society because of their complex personality. Danish HSP Astrid reported that they know that HSPs are not socially relevant and tend to ignore this reality (Cooper, quoted from 2015). Zeff said that most of the social value enhances the low self-image of HSPs. Zeff found that the sensitivity of HSPs was minor and that HSPs may be overwhelmed by society and may feel aggressive behavior, time constraints, the mood of others, and competition. As an example, Aron reported that HSP was misunderstood and looked distant when it tried to include emotions. For example, the

HSP was afraid to make false statements and try to correct perceived injustices. Cooper found that many of the current population view HSPs as neurotic rather than shy or sensitive. As a result, Cooper argued that recognizing the sensitivity of HSPs does not mean that other HSP properties have value or accept them.

Zeff stated that non-HSPs benefit from HSP education on physiological properties. Besides, educating the public reduces HSP's automated response and requires participation in the mirroring of non-HSP behavioral traits compared to others. Zeff noted that HSPs could not control social judgment, but they do not have to feel inferior and can control emotional responses.

Adler (1933/2005) reported that feelings of inadequacy could lead to depression and other psychological problems. According to Jonsson, Grim, and Kjellgren (2014), "it is important to find appropriate treatment options for this group because sensitive individuals tend to have more physiological and cerebral problems than others." Adler (1933/2005) recommended raising public awareness as a movement to heal mental health.

Mistaken Beliefs

Ansbacher found that the psychology of an individual must convey the belief that all psychological insights originated from the individual (quoted from Udchic, 1984). According to Udchic, Adler has developed a lifestyle analysis tool that identifies false beliefs in individuals (that is, myths created and practiced through personal values). These beliefs (learned before age 5) included, for example, attitudes, prejudice, self-assessment, and world-assessment. For example, the misconception is that the world is dangerous, the world is not safe, or the world is challenging and may require competition. False beliefs arise from childhood interpretations that continue into adulthood. Udchic advertised that his childhood beliefs had matured and time-tested for reliability based on his lifestyle. Adler believed that courage to be imperfect was a positive sign, as one did not want to be better than the other due to low feelings. According to Overholser in 2010, Adler has discovered that overcompensation is a protective mechanism that can affect personal development and potentially lead to mental illness. Overholser believed that Adler's psychological approach would help assess the client's lifestyle and reverse inferior emotions and false beliefs. Powers and Griffith (1987) reported that personal psychology encouraged therapists to learn about past restrained experiences testing individual value systems. Besides, behavior patterns are revealed by remembering and rehearsing selected memories that are felt deep within the soul. As an example, Adler argued that revealing childhood memory showed how a child's view of life shifted to adulthood. Besides, Adrian therapists identify beliefs that are valuable, false, and require reformulation.

Adlerian therapists identify early childhood beliefs by studying first childhood memory (Mosak & Di Pietro, 2006). Old memories Use different types of psychological analysis to assess an individual's mental health. According to Mosak and Di Pietro (2006), psychoanalytical instruments included the Minnesota Polymorphic Personality. Inventory (MMPI), Rorschach inkblot test, subject perception test (TAT), and projection test. They said Karl Jung had developed a projection technique called the Word

Association Method. Word association methods included word stimuli and immediate word responses.

A more sophisticated projection technique, known as first mnemonics, could be used anytime, anywhere, (quoted by Mosak & Di Pietro, 2006). Besides, Mosak and Di Pietro highlighted how new memory analysis (ER) exposed the personal value of customers created at a younger age. Moreover, the emergency room can predict behavioral patterns, movements from the past to the present, and decipher future-oriented goals. Carlson, in 2006, reported that an eagle therapist used ER analysis to reveal beliefs from an individual's ethical belief system. For example, these beliefs represented the actions of individuals who preowned to treat themselves and belong to the world. In particular, the emergency room has revealed the motives, strengths, and weaknesses of individual behavior. Using the ER method, an eagle therapist asks the client to recall memories.

After regaining consciousness, the client thinks about how he sees men, women, and the world. The purpose of the emergency room was to reveal childhood memory and analyze it to understand better the client's necessary attitude to life (Pomeroy & Clark, 2015). Pomeroy and Clark reported that they believed that Adler, if one or more areas are missing or insufficient, the person does not feel the whole thing and performs less integrated functions. By using the early memory of therapy, counselors and clients can gain insights from previously undiscovered childhood perspectives and allow individuals to recreate false beliefs from adult interpretations. Pomeroy and Clark added that as early memory becomes apparent, three more questions will consider how he or she sees men, women, and the world. The purpose of the emergency room was to reveal childhood memory and analyze it to better understand the client's necessary attitude to life (Pomeroy & Clark, 2015). Pomeroy and Clark reported that they believed that Adler "if one or more areas are missing or insufficient, the person does not feel the whole thing and performs less integrated functions."). By using the early memory of therapy, counselors and clients can gain insights from previously undiscovered childhood perspectives and allow individuals to recreate false beliefs from adult interpretations. Pomeroy and Clark added that there are three more questions (men, women, the world) that when early memory becomes apparent, treatment analysis allows for unique recognition. As a result, Pomeroy and Clark argue that: "As a projection technique, early memory provides a simple means of assessing the quality level of self-efficacy." Pomeroy and Clark said Adler understood that if an individual were likely to face challenges in adulthood, the consequences would be that individual's self-efficacy. Self-efficacy included emotional, professional, and social balance. In the case of HSPs, self-efficacy can increase trust in all areas of life.

Psychic Development

Aron encouraged HSPs to redefine highly sensitive personality traits. Confidence has expanded our insight into the impact of personal and professional relationships. Aron wanted the HSP to see their unique sensitivity as a personal blessing. Aron's general account of HSP self-awareness and self-care included self-assessment tests, checklists, and review techniques to reveal sensory perception. Aron recommended reformulating past negative experiences to promote trust. Aron believed that confidence leads to the ability to deal with excessive arousal, enrich the mind and spirit, and give discernment to counseling or drug management. Aron's technique included self-calmness through refreshment and relaxation. Aron also recommended that HSP avoid self-insult and apologize for the actions of others. Self-care helps HSPs to learn empathy.

Phobia and depression can occur in the case of HSP if the HSP does not recognize hypersensitivity of personality, anxiety, stress, obsessive-compulsive disorder. In addition to Aron's recommendations for self-care, mindfulness, and grounding techniques, in addition to Adrian's practice, overstimulation can improve mental health symptoms. Aron encouraged HSPs to think carefully, instantly, and consciously. As an example, Aron reported that conscious awareness provided HSPs with the opportunity to redefine negative thoughts and situations. Aron explained that conscious awareness is like confronting fear through mindfulness.

CHAPTER 3: PRACTICING MINDFULNESS

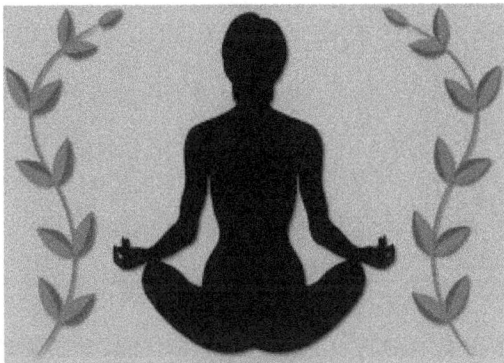

Mindfulness

Soons et al. (2010) discovered that while practicing an eight-week mindfulness meditation program, HSP experienced overwhelming stress, social anxiety, and reduced depression. Also, HSP enhanced emotional empathy, self-acceptance, personal growth, and the ability to transcend. Diana (2014) hypothesized that during the practice of mindfulness, they would get used to the sounds of the body and mind. Through the course of mindfulness, Diana has suggested that people can change thoughts, which ultimately can change emotions. For example, people are beginning to understand that thoughts and feelings are temporary. In short, fluid information forms a flexible mind.

One of the most significant benefits of HSP mindfulness practice is its ability to filter negative energy (rather than absorb it). For example, HSPs can think of an invisible protective shield around their body as a form of self-protection. Similarly, in 2014 Orloff viewed visualization as a technique that HSP's can use to protect from emotional energy. As an example, you can imagine a white light shield or mirror where the HSP is around your body. Another example of visualization during a remarkably deadly encounter, a person would imagine a wild tiger or gorilla patroling the HSP personal space. Diana added that the practice of mindfulness involves choosing to accept overwhelming distractions as a temporary sensation rather than distracting them from infecting individuals with negative energies.

It was HSPs to process more information with intense emotions. Therefore, HSPs are more susceptible to negative emotions that cause anger, fatigue, stress, anxiety, and depression. Aron (2015) recommended that HSPs practice emotional regulation (like mindfulness). To promote emotional regulation, Aron proposed improving the ability of HSPs to:

• Accept your feelings.

• Do not be ashamed of them.

• Believe that you are doing as well as others.

• Believe that bad feelings do not last long.

• Suppose there is hope-after all, you can do something about your destructive emotions.

Confidence and Social Concern

Markowitz (2015b) reports that HSPs tend to feel the physical and emotional pain of others. Markowitz urged the HSP to be very aware of the problem and desire to heal others. In other words, Markowitz suggested that the HSP create a safe and healthy boundary and take care of itself so that it does not try to save others. As a result of self-care practices, HSPs begin to minimize fatigue while maintaining compassion and the ability to empower others to realize their full potential in society.

Orloff (2014) suggested that HSPs can perceive group emotions as they interact with groups (employees, crowds, social events, etc.). For example, according to Zeff (2004), joyful, negative, angry, and sad feelings are absorbed by HSPs, strengthening them. Positive energy enables the HSP to flourish, and negative energy empties, attacks, and damages the HSP. Orloff found that moving at least 20 feet from a negative person reduced the intensity of the empathic response.

Orloff (2014) used the term energy vampire to describe people who exude highly empathetic and positive individuals. When the HSP is about energy vampires, Orloff recommended that the HSP focus on breathing. Orloff encouraged slow, focused inhalation and exhalation, centered on the HSP, and served as a grounding technique. For example, if the HSP focuses on inhaling and exhaling rather than holding your breath, the HSP can visualize the exhalation of negative energy in other people. Besides, the stress of exhaling calms down and prevents emotional fatigue.

Healthy Boundaries

Ward (2012) reported that realistic and healthy limits support HSP self-sufficiency. Besides, healthy boundaries created a safe space and protected emotional energy. He explained, "Understand who you are and what you need, enforce them by setting specific boundaries to recognize your needs, producing results, and acting accordingly." An example of a safe line of demarcation is the agreed deadline when someone requests to help someone. The key to effective separation is to produce reliable results when others do not respect the agreement. Ward believed that healthy limits help create respect, reduce drama, and prevent victim's emotions.

Sand (2016) and Zeff (2004) found that HSPs need to exercise the ability to say no to others through informative and caring answers. Sand (2016) suggested ending conversations like this: "I do not want to end an exciting conversation, but if we continue when we aren't feeling tired." Sand discovered that expressing his thoughts, feelings, and restrictions can help HSPs protect themselves from fatigue. Orloff and Cooper said that "no" is a complete sentence, and no further explanation is necessary if enforced limits predetermined. Zeff found that HSPs are toxic when they suppress information too much, suggesting that they improve practical executive skills in coping with anger, frustration, and frustrating emotions.

Grounding and Nature

Chevalier and Sinatra (2011) found that grounding is a therapeutic tool to reduce a person's response to emotional stress, anxiety, depression, and panic. Chevalier and

Sinatra have shown that grounding techniques include physically standing and lying to connect to the ground. It means that grounding balances the biological nervous system and enhances relaxation. For example, grounding is placing bare feet on the floor for at least 30 minutes. Desirable natural contact includes moist grass, dunes, or wet soil. As a result, the electrons are transmitted through the natural components of Earth and absorbed by the human body. Chevalier and Sinatra said that these electrons promote changes in ANS, regulate sleep patterns and circadian rhythms (physiological cycles of drowsiness and awakening), and improve overall health.

Relaxation

Sand (2016) reports that many relaxation activities can follow through, giving sensitive

HSPs a sense of well-being. The possible actions are:

- Spend on animals.
- Kayaking, sunbathing, weighing in a hammock, working in the garden, arranging flowers.
- (Participate in) Sports, yoga, walking, and meditation practice.
- Read poems and inspirational quotes.
- I love spending time with loved ones and children.
- At night, put a fragrant oil diffuser next to the bed.
- It was outdoors using a sound machine that mimics the elements of nature outdoors.
- Ep Soak your body in Epsom salt or fragrance bath.
- (Regulate) Plan pedicures, manicures, and massages.

- (Perceive)Pain Acupuncture or chiropractic pain and stress healing (Aron, 1996; Cooper, 2015; Sand, 2016; Zeff, 2004).

Aron (1996), Cooper (2015), Sand (2010/2016), and Zeff (2004) recommend spending more than 2 hours a day on HSP to reduce pressure, restore emotional energy, and reduce physical and mental fatigue. Orloff (2014) found that after a busy day's work or after contact with many people, taking baths or showers washed away unnecessary energy. Sand (2016) continues to recommend hobbies such as art, journaling, and dance.

Exercise and Nutrition

To relieve stress, Zeff (2004) and Cooper (2015) encouraged HSPs to take vitamins, avoid processed foods, prepare natural snacks and meals, weekly exercise, and extended sleep. Zeff also recommended changing the bedroom to a womb-like environment. For example, the HSP room should be out of the way of electronics, but it should contain quiet, soothing noise (fans, humidifiers, air conditioners, etc.). Zeff recommended that HSPs adhere to their sleep schedule and do not expose them to bright light when sleeping.

Discussion

Susceptible people are often accused or misdiagnosed for mental disorders. Currently, non-HSPs need to enlighten on highly sensitive personality traits. Aron found that HSP was misdiagnosed and concerned as depression, anxiety, or neurosis. Besides, the HSP population may not be aware of the sensitivity that causes untreated problems with low self-esteem of HSP. HSPs may feel unreliable, emotionally unresponsive, inferior, misunderstood, underestimated, confused, subordinate, lonely, or isolated. Because of the cognitively specific processing style of highly sensitive individuals, many therapists may not be aware that symptoms of anxiety, stress, or depression may result from the processing of details.

Aron suggested that 30-50% of healthcare professionals have difficulty identifying, understanding, and treating HSP clients. Also, these relationship difficulties can affect the closest relationship with the HSP's parents, children, and spouse. For example, if the HSP requires at least 2 hours of downtime per day, the non-HSP may be dissatisfied or discriminated against by the HSP and maybe lazy, selfish, or withdrawn.

In 2007, Northwestern University revealed how the misdiagnosis of human personality traits in the pharmaceutical industry had opened the door to the diagnosis and prescription of pharmaceuticals. Northwestern University continues: "Psychiatrists claim that the boundaries between usual shyness and social anxiety disorder are clearly defined, but Lane repeatedly confuses her, risking patients overdiagnosis and unnecessary and sometimes harmful treatment. Misdiagnosis can further destroy the life of the HSP and cause further confusion. Unethical misdiagnosis of the HSP can cause severe damage to the HSP. They are giving and promoting withdrawal from society. Understanding the personality traits of HSP through individual psychological lenses helps reduce misdiagnosis and promotes well-being. Also, the lack of HSP training Can lead to misunderstandings and affect social benefits. A better understanding of HSP susceptibility is essential for counseling HSP individuals and their families.

The mental health profession requires HSP training and awareness to correctly assess and advise 30% of HSP minorities. Knowledge is vital in the field of mental health, as ethical guidelines are imposed on mental health professionals to protect clients and therapists from potential harm. Psychiatrists do not want to risk the license to rescind or the complaint being filed with the Board because the features of HSP are not well known. For example, Sand explained that a therapist could give HSP clients homework, visit crowded places, build relationships with strangers, and overcome social fears. Sand has suggested that this is a dangerous exposure to an environment that is overly irritating and may increase the overwhelming fear of HSP clients. As a result, HSP clients become increasingly uncomfortable and afraid to connect with other users. Also, the therapist may misdiagnose the client for social anxiety or agoraphobia (separation of social interaction) or refer the HSP to a psychiatrist for drug management to help the HSP crowd and social anxiety. You can minimize your fear. Sand concludes that the therapist was untrained and unable to assess and identify the characteristics of HSPs. As a result, clients may experience additional stress, panic, anxiety, and unwanted and potentially harmful drug management. After all, HSPs only wanted the ability to deal with unwanted energy and the negative emotions of others. Aron reported that HSPs could benefit significantly from treatments to restore normality when dealing with overwhelming relationships in work, connections, and health.

Impact on Practice

In 2015 Abramson, explained that people belong to and must contribute to society. Regarding Adler's notion of social interests, Abramson proposed that "the intertwining of human and group happiness. In contrast, the lack of sense of belonging increases the importance of inferiority. As a result, lack of attribution can undermine community interest, delay HSP's contribution to society, and impede the achievement of HSP's purpose in life.

Education

From a social interest perspective, the purpose of training non-HSPs is to generate general awareness of the characteristics of HSPs and an understanding of HSP's unique gifts. Education efforts include community workshops, individual and family HSP retreats, and components of psychoeducation for personal and family therapy.

This knowledge helps practitioners build relationships, promote mutual respect, and perceived equality with potential HSPs, as it allows professionals to understand the complexity and nature of the personality traits of HSPs. Due to the limited research on HSPs, there is no "medical remedy" for this sensory processing property. Considering this, improving treatment options for HSPs and supporting HSP-specific emotional sensitivity can make mental health prophylactic and ethical.

When the client chooses a treatment, the first recommendation is that all therapists consider the potential of HSP clients. Helping specialists can consistently include HSP surveys in the assessment process. The HSP self-test identifies feelings or features that have overwhelming, inability to concentrate, fatigue, stress, anxiety, or depression. As a result, the HSP self-test assessment tool introduces, assesses, and discloses the properties and characteristics of HSPs. If you are an identified HSP, you can now be empowered, understood, accepted, evaluated, and confident.

In contrast, without identifying the characteristics of HSPs, clients can remain anomalous and misunderstood. The therapist was able to find a free and sensitive survey for therapists. After responding to the questionnaire, the therapist was able to prepare and educate HSPs and identify treatment plans, including identifying false beliefs.

As I said, false belief refers to the values and ideas established in childhood (Mosak & Di Pietro, 2006). The use of emergency rooms helps HSPs identify the causes of false beliefs that hinder their self-esteem and their feelings about how they are observed and lived in the world. Useful According to Aron (2004), the treatment task is to distinguish the effects of such difficulties in childhood from those that do not require treatment. Even a typical effect of properties.

Early memory leads HSPs to reveal and understand lifestyle beliefs, attitudes, and beliefs about how HPS perceives men, women, and the world. Therapists encourage HSPs to reveal visual events from childhood (before age 10) and explain this memory through narrative explanations. The therapist asks the HSP to describe the most precise moment in mind. Next, the therapist asks where the HSP is feeling the body at that moment. The therapist explains that the potential importance of this emergency room is related to the position of the client's life in its memory. The priority assigned to the emergency room is an interpretation that may reveal false beliefs. Emergency rooms indicate false beliefs and how these beliefs affect clients as adults. The therapist tries to pinpoint childhood beliefs and asks clients how they behave differently as adults. This approach allows clients to re-adjust adult self-awareness and social outlook. After collecting five emergency rooms from customers Tom, Mosak, and Di Pietro (2006), when we asked the following question, we identified the topic and pattern within the emergency room.

- How does he get what he wants?

- How do other people treat him in difficult times?

- How does he see men?

- How does he look at a woman?

- How does he know the world?

- How does he treat life?

After collecting three to five emergency rooms, the therapist was able to adapt and use the previous questions to gain potential insights and interpretations for clients and therapists. Clients and therapists can use the information to reveal patterns in the context of social interaction and relationships. When trends and false beliefs indicate, clients and therapists can engage in a reformulation process to disrupt HSP's previous self-ironing thoughts, feelings, and reactions.

Therapeutic intervention after the identification of HSP clients, educated about specific personality traits, and false beliefs bring out, the therapist and the client can develop an HSP self-care plan. At this point in the treatment process, the therapist incorporates various interventions and techniques into the treatment environment. Responses can bespeak to the specific interests and skills of the customer.

As described by Soons et al. (2010), Mindfulness practices help HSPs relieve stress, social anxiety, and depression. The therapist teaches mindfulness skills during the therapy session and encourages the HSP to stay in the present moment. The goal is to increase self-acceptance and promote personal growth. For example, HSP clients practice using mindfulness techniques to coordinate emotions. The therapist can teach the client to use Allon's (1996) suggestions to adjust emotions. HSP clients can be encouraged to accept non-embarrassing emotions and understand their ability to deal with intense emotions and feelings.

Mindfulness practices can increase confidence in false beliefs. Therapists can include an emergency room in their mindfulness practice and self-confidence by requiring clients to relate to childhood memories. Customers can transfer memories to adult's behaviors. Besides, the therapist can facilitate conversations about HSP's strengths (or gifts). The therapist can teach clients to develop emotional and physical self-confidence through self-comfort, reformulation of false beliefs, and relaxation techniques. Conscious awareness of mindfulness allows HSP clients to face fear and create an understanding that they need to hear rather than feel right or wrong.

Daily journal tasks help HSPs identify and redefine emotional responses. The client raises to record his perception of stressful moments when he feels overwhelmed. If the HSP client is aware of the opinions and ideas related to stressful situations, the client can begin setting appropriate limits. Healthy boundaries can create a safe space and protect the emotional energy of HSPs. Healthy boundaries include the ability to say no and the ability to release emotions and claims. Therapists can mitigate healthy boundaries by rehearsing meaningful conversations and building the ability to set client trust and boundaries.

The therapist can ask the client to schedule at least two hours of rest to recharge their emotional energy. This downtime could include the grounding of Chevalier and Sinatra and natural technology (i.e., 30 minutes of physical connection to Earth). Rest may consist of various mitigation techniques tailored to the specific needs of the HSP. According to Zeff (2004) and Cooper (2015), HSPs need to manage exercise and a healthy diet. When people exercise, they release endorphins, reduce stress, and improve sleep. Therapists can incrementally develop health and wellness goals to drive HSP clients into general well-being. To remain confident, encouraged, and acknowledged, the therapist can help HSP clients to participate in several different lessons. For example, a customer can do one of the following weekly tasks:

• Investigate information about HPS and train therapists.

• Identify a list of HSP strengths.

• Watch assigned HSP YouTube videos and discussed them during the session.

• Sign up for the HSP social media website.

• Feelings and thoughts in the diary about the emergency room.

• Express emotions using creative techniques such as drawing, painting, and painting.

• Have a music text that identifies your current feelings.

• After mindfulness practice, participate in daily mindfulness practice and diary.

• Create a wish list (or bucket list) and discuss it in a meeting.

• Plan your diet and exercise.

If clients participate in the treatment as mentioned above processes (i.e., identification of HSP features and false beliefs, therapeutic interventions, and self-care practices), this will reduce obstruction and increase interest in social activities and relationships. Adler described his attitude toward life and social sentiment as the ability to "see with others, hear with others, feel with others" (quoted from Ansbacher & Ansbacher, 1956). HSPs already seem to work at a deeper level of empathy than the average person. If the HSP can complete the treatment process and appreciate the gift, it can manage the social interactions. At the end of the treatment process, HSP clients may be willing to participate in activities and new social relationships. Homework of social interests include:

• Bring your dessert to your new neighbor.

• Participate in social work events.

• Volunteer for community events.

• Visit care facilities or places of interest.

Conclusion

To improve the quality of life of HSPs, therapists can do a lot. First, educating the public and therapists will improve non-HSP understanding of specific strengths and talents associated with HSPs. Second, the therapist should be aware that HSPs may participate in the treatment process. That is, HSPs can enter the treatment process due to symptoms that can be confused with another diagnosis. The therapist should eliminate the possibility of using HSP before assigning a diagnosis (or misdiagnosis) to an HSP client. When a knowledgeable therapist treats HSP clients, HSPs can far exceed current expectations for happiness, health, and emotional health.

CHAPTER 4: SURVIVAL GUIDE

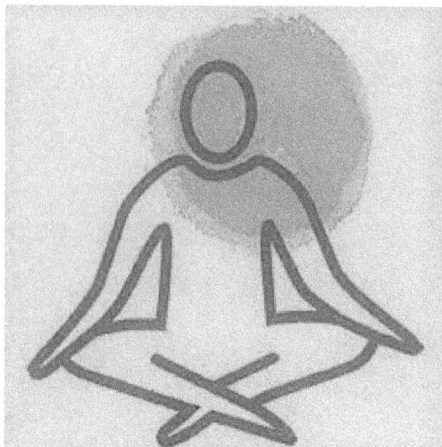

Empath's Survival Guide

I provide Empath's Survival Guide as a resource for the relevant sensitive souls to find understanding and acceptance in a world often harsh, heartless, and delicate. In it, we challenge the status quo and create new normality to show sensitivity anywhere in the spectrum. There is nothing "wrong" about being sensitive. You are trying to understand what is "right" for you. In this book, accompanying audio programs, Empaths essential tools, and Empaths workshops, I would like to create a community of support to help you find your tribe and shine real. I want to support the movement of people who respect their sensibility. Welcome to the circle of love! My message to you is one of hope and acceptance. We encourage you to accept the gifts and do your best to empathize with them.

How Does Empathy Manifest, And Which Areas Affect Our Lives?

Empathy can exist in the following aspects of everyday life. Many people with empathy skills have seen me overwhelmed, tired, and exhausted before learning practical skills to deal with their sensibility. People often diagnosed with agoraphobia, chronic fatigue, fibromyalgia, migraine, chronic pain, allergies, and adrenal exhaustion (a type of burnout syndrome). At an emotional level, anxiety, depression, and panic attacks can occur. Many sympathizers rely on alcohol, drugs, food, sex, shopping, and other habits to paralyze their susceptibility. Overeating is common. You can accidentally use the menu to ground yourself. The additional pad protects negative energy and can quickly become overweight—relationship, love, and sex. Sympathizers may unknowingly engage with a toxic partner, leading to anxiety, depression, or illness. As a person with empathy, you may easily give your mind to narcissists and other unavailable people. They love and expect others, but not always. You can absorb your partner's stress and emotions, such as anger and depression, by merely interacting and romancing. Finally, you can learn how to build healthy relationships without being overwhelmed, expel toxic people from your life, or set definite limits.

Sympathetic parents often find themselves overwhelmed and exhausted by the intensive need to raise children because they tend to absorb the emotions and pain of their children. Also, empathetic children can overcome their sensitivity. Their parents need specialized training to help these children and promote their gifts.

Job is the other overwhelming area. If you are sensitive, you may feel overwhelmed by energy vampires at work, but you do not know how to set limits. You can learn to be centered and replenished in a work environment where there may be little privacy, or there may be excessive irritation—outstanding cognitive ability. You can make your sensitivity more intuitive, feel the energy of people, and be open to prediction, animal communication, and dreams. Over time, you'll learn how to empower yourself with these empathic skills. Benefits and challenges of empathy. Being empathetic have both advantages and challenges. Typical uses of understanding I am grateful to be a compassionate person and thankful for the blessings my sensibility gives me every day. I love being intuitive, feeling the energy flow of the world, reading people, and experiencing the richness of being so open to life and nature.

We have many excellent qualities for those with whom we have sympathies. We have a great heart and instinct to help those in need and those who are not wealthy. We are dreamers and idealists. We are passionate, sincere, creative, emotional, compassionate, and able to see the big picture. We understand the feelings of others and can be loyal friends and friends. We are intuitive, spiritual, and feel the energy. We naturally have a special appreciation and a sense of comfort.

Sympathetic people often resonate with nature, plants, forests, and gardens. We love water. Even if you soak hot water in a uterine bath or live near the sea or river, you will invigorate. We deal with animal rescue and animal communication, feeling connected with our animal companions.

Common Challenges to Empathize

When you start to face challenges and feel more comfortable than empathy, you enjoy all the right things. The common problems I have seen with my patients and workshop participants are:

You Are Becoming Overstimulated

As a person with empathy, you often feel like a raw nerve ending, and you burn up quickly because you don't have the same defenses as others. If you don't have enough time to replenish and relax daily, you can suffer from the toxic effects of overstimulation and sensory overload. Absorb the stress and negativity of others. Sometimes empathetic people may not be able to distinguish your feelings and emotional differences from those of others. It can cause a variety of physical and psychological symptoms, ranging from pain to fear. We feel things hard. You may not be able to watch violent or stimulating movies about people or animals because of the atrocity that aches. You can bear the burden of the world and feel the pain of others and witness the news.

Experience emotional and social hangover. If there are too many people, feelings are too loud, or if you are sensitive, you may feel hypersensitivity and discomfort for a long time after the event. The world seems so overwhelming that empathizes can either isolate themselves or move away from them. As a result, others may find you uncomfortable, but in fact, they scan your surroundings very carefully to make sure it is safe. You can also freeze fake people who can report reluctance. However, this is a protective device.

Experience is emotional burnout. The downside of being very considerate is that people get together at you to tell the story of their lives. Since childhood, there have been invisible signs that "I can help you." As a result, empathize must set clear boundaries for others and cannot "give away."

They are addressing increased sensitivity to light, odor, taste, touch, temperature, and noise. Loud sounds and bright lights are painful to many empathetic people and me. They penetrate our bodies and shock them. Keep your ears closed when the ambulance drives. Also, fireworks cannot explode. They scare me as a scary dog reacts. Sympathizers have improved startle response and respond very quickly to intensive sensory input. Strong odors and chemicals such as exhaust gases and perfumes give us discomfort, allergies, and choking sensations. We are sensitive to extreme temperatures and may dislike air conditioning. Our bodies are supplied with energy or discharged by severe weather such as thunderstorms, gusts, or snowfall. Many sympathizers are excited by the bright full moon. Others are excited about it.

Express your needs in an intimate relationship. If you live in the same room or share a bed with someone, there are needs related to empathy. You may need a different place and a separate foundation to feel comfortable. As empathy, it's essential to talk with your partner about your needs.

Understanding is not "irritability." They have gifts, but they need to learn to deal with their sensitivity.

Prosper as Empathy

In this book, you will learn skills to master the challenges and improve the many benefits of empathy. Society may suggest that you are "more sensitive" and "harder," but I encourage you to develop your sensitivity and stay with them. Being an empathetic person is a great asset when you learn to deal with them. You are crazy, not "nervous," hypochondriatic, or vulnerable. You are a great, sensitive person with the talent to need the tools to deal with it.

One of the skills that sensitive people need to learn is how to deal with sensory overload if they become too fast. It can make you tired, anxious, depressed, or sick. You may feel that there is no on / off switch for empathy, as many of us do. That is not true. Here's how to manage your sensitivity rather than being bullied. The world becomes your playground when you feel protected and safe. To gain peace of mind, you need to identify some common factors that cause empathy overload. Start identifying triggers. You can then act quickly to correct the situation.

What makes empathic overload symptoms worse? Fatigue, illness, busy pace, traffic, large numbers of people, noisy environment, large numbers of people, toxic people, conflict, overwork, too cheerful, such as parties and cruises. The feeling of being trapped in a new situation. Any combination of these forces increases empathic overload. So, keep in mind: stress + hypoglycemia = drama and fatigue.

What can improve the symptoms of empathic overuse? When I feel sensory overload, I must slow everything down and disconnect from all stimuli. When it gets so strong, it feels like a flower that has withered and needs to set upright in silence. Then retire to a room with no sound or light, sleep, or meditate to reduce the stimulus and recondition yourself. On days and weekends, when sensory overload is extreme, quarantine may be required from time to time. But during this time, you can take short nature walks and limited trips to get things done. The problem is that often the empathy doesn't see all or all. They are moving in their lives or retreating in a haven in their home. It is advisable to balance this and soften this radical stance so that you do not suffer from excessive loneliness or solitude. Hear your intuition about what you feel is right. Each of us must find a unique way to meet our needs.

Shielding is also an essential skill, recommended to prevent excessive empathy. It's a quick way to protect yourself.

Many sympathizers rely on shields to hide toxic energy while allowing positive free flow. We recommend that you use this skill regularly. If you feel uncomfortable with people, places, or situations, raise the signboard immediately. Use when talking to Energy Vampires at airports, parties, or in a doctor's busy waiting room. Because of the shield, you are in a safe bubble, and you are not out.

Protection Strategy: Protecting Visualization for Empathy

Imagine a beautiful shield made of white or pink light that, when relaxed, surrounds your body and extends a few inches away. This shield protects you from harmful, stress, toxicity, and invasion. You are feeling focused, happy, and energetic under the protection of this shield. This shield blocks negativeness, but at the same time, you can feel positive and loving. Get used to the feeling of security that protects your body. Having people who have empathy is a valuable skill. You can visualize the protection whenever you suspect that it is absorbing the energy of others.

In addition to the shield, empathic self-care means eating well every day to minimize stress. Also, specific actions are body and soul balms. These include taking time for rest, contacting positive people, being in nature, soaking in water to get rid of negative energy, vampire meditation of power, and exercise. Determine your intention to incorporate these forms of self-care into your daily life regularly. I also firmly believe in personal rituals and meditations for people with empathy to ground themselves, such as:

Grounding and The Power of Grounding

Grounding is a method of connecting yourself to the energy of the earth. Of course, it's ideal to go barefoot, but you can also use it in the lawn garden. Or you can get a full effect by placing your whole body towards the ground. I love resting on the sea and looking up at the sky. Earth's energy is medicine for stressed people, especially those who have empathy and empathy. When you touch the earth, you can start healing from your feet and whole body. High-density reflexology massage and acupuncture points on the soles of the feet are activated by walking and massaging barefoot, which is especially useful in the case of grounding stress. Your feet can convey the healing of the earth to your others.

However, if you are unable to be in nature, you can use the following visualization techniques at home, at work, or in social situations. If you don't have a private room, you can always take a break and go outside or go to the bathroom for a few minutes. Practice this visualization, decompress, and return to the center.

Protective Strategy

If you are overworked, anxious, or feel anxious, give yourself some quiet time to reduce your stimulation level. As a sensitive person, it helps you to be alone and to relax and recharge. Close the door, turn off your computer and phone. Then sit in a comfortable position and take a few deep breaths to relax your body. You will feel calm and relaxed while the tension releases. Just breathe and relax. When they come up, let them pass like clouds in the sky. Don't stick to them. Focus on inhaling slowly and then exhaling. Feel the tranquility and stress that remains in your body.

Imagine a large, strong trunk with a large tree in this quiet interior, extending from head to toes across the center of your body. Take a moment to feel its strength and vitality. Then imagine how the roots of a tree grow from the bottom of the foot, heart on the ground, and go deep and deep. Stick your roots in Mother Earth and stabilize your empathy.

Rooting for yourself provides the inner strength to focus and protect your life, which can quickly happen as an empathizer, becomes overwhelming. If you slowly open your eyes, you will feel the ground repeatedly. Go back to the room and use this ground visualization to make sure you can lock yourself in when you fall.

Grounding is an essential skill to keep you healthy and empathetic. Focusing on your feet, not your fear or overwhelming feeling, is a quick way to focus. (A foot massage also works mysteriously to get you out of your head into your body). Regularly practice this and other medications to reduce sensory overload.

Blessing to Empathize

When you start your journey, remember that your presence, your sweetness, the gentle appreciation of people, and your life are gifts to you and others. Heal your intuition and sophisticated sensitivity. I want you to rate yourself, your openness, and your ability to feel. Understand how special and perfect you are. If you see yourself, you relate to your inner wholeness and depth. Then you can enjoy empathy. That's the point. Not everyone understands you, but it's okay. You can also find them by looking for related spirits. It's a beautiful connection.

You are a pioneer during the development of human consciousness and as a sympathizer. The sacred responsibility is to be the empathy that demands more from you than merely stopping isolation. It is essential to learn how to be overwhelmed so that you can fully exercise your power in the world. You are the forefront pioneer of a new way for humanity. They are generations of sensitive-people who welcome compassion and kindness. They are an essential beginning for society to become a more central and more intuitive place. For others, you can emulate empathy-sensitive and robust methods.

I am excited to help you deal with your empathic abilities and sensibilities and show you how you can use them for your personal and better interests. I've learned to respect myself as empathy, an incredible overall sense, and I hope you will also appreciate the gift of understanding. Use the information in this article to help you be more personal than ever. To start your journey, I offer you the following confirmations:

Positive Empathy

I pledge to treat everyone lovingly while respecting their sensitivity, empathizing, and exploring what it means to accept a gift.

CHAPTER 5: MENTAL HEALTH TO REDUCE STRESS AND FIND YOUR SENSE OF SELF

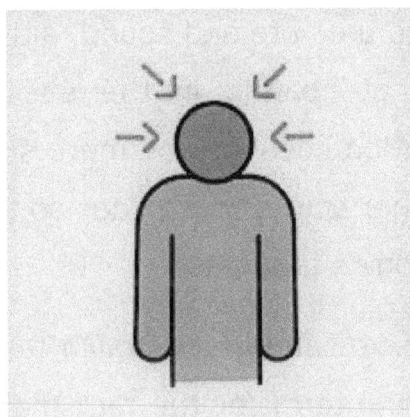

First, meditation is the key to opening your mental capacity.

Definition

It is the ability to see an image or image-like vision through the mind's eye (the third eye). The third eye is in the middle of the forehead between the forehead and the eyebrows. Clairvoyants are sometimes called seekers.

Clear hearing (SOUND) is the ability to hear sounds and voices through the eyes of the mind. It is the ear of your thoughts that "listens" to the vote and sound, although it is the area of hearing in the ear. Also, its sophistication seems to be more subtle than that of other spirits and guides so that it can decipher one's thoughts.

A distinct sensation/feel (touch/taste/smell) is the actual term for the fact that you can feel psychologically through physical sensations. It is a particular "knowledge" that lies deep inside you. Clairsentients can also make physical contact or feel like people or what they perceive. (A deviation from this ability in the strong sense is called empathy.)

Your intuition brings all the mental sensations. If you do not know the image or sound you received, you can rely on your intuition to guide you. You can ask if your interpretation is correct, and you will feel intuition-yes or no strength of the gastric cavity through the solar plexus.

Universal Roll

Learn Deja Vu, sync, coincidence, and how to test the Universe yourself!

You will also experience soul signatures, vectors, ethics, and energy vampires.

"I want a spiritual light here.

I have a clear and perfect channel.

I am love, and I am light. "

Awakens Mental and Mental Abilities and Spiritual Consciousness

First, we are all somewhat psychological. We can all use supernatural powers. Some people don't accept their skills. For many, it takes time to blossom and realize your unique potential. You really need to recognize the potential of your consciousness, and most importantly, Practice continuously and use these skills as often as possible. Increasing the level of vibration will allow you to accept feelings. It can bring off through practice and meditation. In addition to my spiritual awareness, I have found in my experience that you are growing more spiritually. It seems that the two are holding hands.

At least when you receive the message, some people in the Mental Awareness division don't work well, but you may have to use it to find it. I've heard a lot of divination, but I've seen this ability and awareness come naturally. Since they recognize their abilities and recognize them almost immediately after birth, they can be called "natural sellers."

These special people can always use their talents. In some cases, this ability is so strong that it needs to be closed. These people may need to learn how to turn off and control skills when they don't need them or when they need to use them. I need the ability. And it's also what we all heard when we suddenly acquired these new skills after a tragic personal event. Perhaps something near the accident, a lightning strike (if you survived), or death can raise your awareness.

In the rest of us, there are practices. Faith and dedication are the two main components. So, when you think, engage, train, meditate and become more open to your presence in spiritual strength. It is crucial to protect yourself when you open yourself (that is when you meditate or read other people). Please say the above prompt before opening. It saves you and opens you for a reception.

Surround yourself with white light, beautiful visualizations, and everything else that acts as an individual.

"When light rivet and directed, like a telescope or microscope, we can see something beyond the boundaries of our senses. Love is in focus. It's time to be oriented, to learn something about people and things which are not possible without love. We know something about ourselves; yes, Love expands our horizons.

People meditated on watching TV, dreaming in class, and zoning themselves on their way home. Don't say you can't because you can. Whether it's a deeper level of meditation or not, you can do it. You can go as deep as you like with practice. However, it is enough to meditate for 15-30 minutes a day and cleanse your heart. Whenever you need a "breather," you can do it well and meditate. Many people misunderstand meditation.

First, most people think you need to clear your mind

It is not entirely possible or necessary. For that, you can only change the level of consciousness. The background noise cannot always bend off. Play new age music to calm down and relax. You can hear the traffic and people just keep going.

People did this many time with noise, and it's possible. Meditation is the door to your other senses-the the sixth sense. First, takes a deep breath through your nose and mouth. Positive IN, negative OUT. Just relax and breathe. Imagine when you are sitting (usually, I don't fall asleep because I must do it). Your body relaxes from every part of the body, from feet to head. Slowly but surely, the meditative "state" is also called the alpha state. You are in a neutral place. It has nothing to do with emotions, people, places, or things.

You can try the following two versions. For example, imagine a place where you feel happy. A beautiful garden with flowers and sea, or just let go of your thoughts and notice. Now, you are a viewer. Share your ideas as if you were an invited viewer.

With one of these techniques, you can see that thinking is going in all directions. Think of yourself and say "escape" and breathe. Don't worry, think carefully about where you need it and adjust. When you have an idea, carefully return to the right path. Don't think! It just returns to visualization or focus, depending on what you do and what you don't. After that, the breathing is short and barely noticeable. Being passive is essential when you are frustrated or upset. Things will improve at the pace you should follow, photos will be sharper, stay in sight longer, and you can track them and get more. If you can sit outside (e.g., sleeping on a bed or wall). Comfortable, liar, it's a good position. But like everything it deserves, it takes time and practice!

Psychological Information Method and Belief

Intuition

We all have clues. It is our little voice deep inside us. Some call it the voice of God. Call it what you want. It will work for you if you listen. All intuitions can only make use to learn to hear them. If you feel deep, you know what will happen next, or do you know you should be walking down one street instead of the other? Your first impression will not mislead you. Whatever your intuition tells you, even if you hear something awful from your intuition, it will be right. It is very likely that your intuition guided you into this situation learned from more horrifying experiences, and kept you away from those more horrifying experiences. Don't doubt it because they fear it and think about what your intuition tells you. Opening and listening to this little voice also open your mind's awareness. Intuition is unique to everyone. The trick is to decipher your thoughts and feelings from your intuition. When you hear something negative, it's not your intuition. Your intuition is not emotional; it informs you in your way. You probably feel something that physically alerts you to danger. You can think from the back, bite your stomach, hear, see, and feel what you can intuitively understand. If you don't think about the message too long, your thoughts can get in the way of your words, completely confusing your intuition from the beginning. Always do with your first feelings and intuition. I cannot stress this enough. Don't doubt it because you are new! "Ah, it's okay. Either way, think first. Either way, give the first impression.

Because mental skills are also related to intuition, and they are almost the same.

Mental Skills

Psychological skills are related to your intuition. Intuition tells you when the message you receive is correct or if you need to dig deeper to convey the message better. It is challenging to separate intuition from your intellectual ability. As it is mentioned, we all have these skills. Some skills may be more reliable than others, but they may not. Decide whether to improve these skills. You need to do the same in perspective, especially if you want to improve your ability to draw and become a dancer.

Skills and Awareness

Another word used in psychic skills is E.S.P. ("Extra Sensory Perception" is the basis of all psychology disciplines. There are physical sensations and psychological sensations or "channels" that react together).

The focus of this class is on perspective, but I think it is vital to study all aspects to reveal different types of mental abilities. It also helps you understand where your strengths are and where you can improve your skills.

What Are Your Strengths?

Everyone has strengths. You will be able to see the pictures immediately during the meditation. And with practice, you will be able to see more photos faster. It takes time and responsibility. I was known for relaxing while meditating. Relaxing makes it more and more challenging to receive messages and pictures. So, you need to start over, meditate, and sharpen my consciousness. You had to do some other work because it was legible. You need to work on clairvoyance (know when your emotions, feelings, and sensations belong to someone.

In some cases, you may be able to "listen" for sounds and voices rather than "see" the photo. Test this to see your strengths. Some people receive information as emotions, while others receive information through things like images, sounds, thoughts, verbal messages, or pure "knowledge." Understanding how to win is fundamental.

Perspective

Perspective is the ability to see an image or image-like vision through the mind's eye (the third eye). The third eye is in the middle of the forehead between the forehead and the eyebrows. Clairvoyants are sometimes called seekers. Information is available in several ways. A big dreamy vision, or a "face" vision that needs to be defined, can look real. The best idea is to write it down immediately without feelings or thoughts.

Some of us use objects such as tarot cards, crystal balls, and candles that correlate with various aspects of the occult field for centuries. These are great tuning buttons on the receiver. It gives us something to focus our consciousness on. It helps us get out of the picture and improve our concentration. Once you are relaxed, these are not needed unless the see-through is required. In many cases, the reader is staring at the universe, not the one they are using. It is a sign that the reader's perspective (and other spiritual gifts) will come.

Clairaudience-Clear Hearing

Clear hearing (SOUND) is the ability to hear sounds and voices through the eyes of the mind. The area where you "listen" is the area of the ear, but it is your third eye that "listens" for voices and sounds. It also seems more subtle than the spirits of other spirits and spirit guides when it comes to elaborate handicrafts with the ability to decipher their thoughts.

It is more subtle than listening loudly. There are quiet sounds that you hear (sounds like "in your head" like thoughts, nothing about emotions). You can listen to current, past, or future distances. You can hear the guide speak to you and other spirits (or mental media skills). Loudness undeniably fits your mental ears.

Clairsentience - Clear-Sensing

The clear sensation is the correct term that can be felt mentally through physical sensations. Clairsentients can reach and feel as if they were that person or something they knew. It is also your inner knowledge and feelings about something upcoming. (This ability is very different from empathy.) The accurate perception is the "mental sponge." Absorbs the entire environment around you and the other you meet your emotions, negativity, positive emotions, etc. You can separate the empathy of another person's body perspective and another person's emotions.

This feature (like other features, but this feature is essential for saving someone else's debris) clears many features. If you want to remove someone else's rubble, you need to use the button. An excellent example of an interruption is the idea that the phone has hung up. If your emotions are too loud, watch the phone hang up. Dress in WHITE LIGHT and ask your guide or angel for help. There are many things you can do to free yourself from the trash of others.

Empathy is the ability to feel the emotions and conditions of other psychologically. At the psychological level, empathy shares the feelings of others and often cannot control them. It is also empathy to feel the "aura" of a person. "He chilled me" is an expression of probing someone's aura. Sympathizers often know the thoughts of others, but they do not read them. It absorbs emotions that reflect the opinions of others. It is also the ability to be sensitive and receptive to external emotional stimuli. Some people call empathy "sensitive."

Emotions are essential feedback, don't be afraid, just understand. If you only know a person's feelings, you can tell them and publish them directly to address the emotions and causes and do something. When they see them, they feel it and release these emotions only once, depending on whether they are wrong. If it gets too big, be sure to wrap yourself in white light. The use of this energy reduction visualization offers various protection measures—the idea of a filter that can capture all energy vibrations that are not yours. But the emotional power behind the intention is that job. Stay away to make the problem worse! You can also work on other levels (if possible) to change your emotional energy.

The transformation of emotional energy into love is compelling. If you imagine stroking the energy field with your eyes, the energy field will also be deformed and balanced.

Clear Smell

It is different from Clairsentience. The feeling of "beyond." It is usually associated with medium combat. Maybe you are looking for someone who has a ghost over there and smells of roses. They talk about it and make sure that this unique scent has a special meaning to those who know it mentally. If you're doing the general mental reading and need to cross on to the subject, you can also have the same spiritual odor for something alive. This ability is not limited to medium vessels. You can even taste it psychologically, not what you feel. What a heart or soul (that is, a cigar, metal, etc.) can taste everything related to that person.

Healing

There are several repair methods. However, in general, recovery means sending energy to others and situations to heal them to their best condition. There are names like Reiki (there are different types of Reiki like Karuna and Rainbow), energy healing, practical healing. For the natural healers, they are incorporated and instantly healed from space, but they also include healing energy. But in most cases, healing powers do not come directly from us. It affects healers, but it affects the universe. Reiki removes the healing energy from the universal life force that reaches the person we heal.

Everyone has strengths here, as well. What are your muscles? "I am a healer. No one can make you a healer. It is the only way to call it. Yet there are different types of treatments. Different people have different healing methods. The Belief that Everything Exists. There is energy, and every person is composed of energy that connects to the other person. Aura before it appears in the body of the "body," Some people claim to appear. For healing aura and sometimes body. When used with love, cosmic energy is free and infinite. When you adapt to love, you adjust to the healing powers of the world. Healing is with the idea of motivating love. It is also tuning/vibration. When you are in the "love" mindset, your pulse will be very close to the waves of the universe. But the most common healing method is to use your mind. I summon the healing and conscious white light of God to fill and wrap me up. When ready, place your hand on the person whom you are treating. Imagine the crown chakra opening and drawing white light from space. After this, imagine that this white light passing through your head, right arm, and right hand. Visualize laser-like energy from the middle of the right palm. Visualize the energy flowing into the worker and the power to pull out the left palm. It's like a long distance. For me, my right hand can feel the heat. It is the body that draws out the energy a baby sucks in a bottle. People extract energy coming from space through. When this tension disappeared, the body received all the power it needed at that time. Next, imagine the strength to return to space. I always wash my hands before and after healing. At times, I imagined energy as a color in response to "feeling." We feel breathless. I used flavors (must be all-natural essential oils!). Healing can take many forms. One of the best ways to get started is to grab a person's foot (with or without socks). I track the breathing of working people-this synchronizes me with their bodies. Then I open the healing energy of the universe. I usually use the crown chakra. You can also use the heart chakra. I like chelating my body from my legs. I start the flow of energy (from the crown chakra to the right palm, from the left palm to the crown chakra).

The sender and my left hand will always be my recipient. I put my right hand behind the person's foot and my left hand on the ankle (by starting with the foot approach, the body should be on the right when facing the head) -releasing energy. I feel a subtle electric impulse in my left hand, waiting for a sense of unity. Then move your left hand to your knee. I send energy from the right side through the person's foot and ankle to the knee and then to the left hand. If you get an electric shock, place your left hand on the person's waist and repeat the above steps. The left-hand moves from size to genitals. Then release your needle, grab the other leg, and try again. I'm always on the same page. I'm not on every side of my body. The right hand always sends. Even if you turn the person over, you will not receive your left hand and will not cross. Once you have completed both feet in the base chakra, train your upper body from one chakra to the next. Finish the top of your head with both hands. If you do not feel a subtle electrical stimulus, release it and rub it together for a short time. Then put your hands back on the person's body.

You don't have to touch anyone. You can do all this a little above. Then rewash your hands. It helps clarify energy. Okay, it's long and probably confusing. Please read this a few times to see if it makes sense. Remember that you work with very subtle emotions and energies. Energy is required when it is cold. (This changes the meaning of coldness and warmth per person!) Your hands get very hot. That is energy. People always comment on my warm hands. Use your intuition again when deciding where to go with a person. Usually, I start with the crown chakra and go to the right. The left side of the body as the healers upstairs because they increased my healing potential, my energy, and my spiritual performance.

Believe

You must believe that when you are alone! This belief felt up in the reading room. It is usually a good read if the actor/client believes in your skills as well. However, if you are unsure, this will be displayed, and your gift will decline in the long run. It's difficult to grow yourself without believing in yourself or thinking about the skills you want to develop. Remember that not everyone who comes to you has the same beliefs as you. If not, some will start showing you. Some come to prove that you are right but make it very difficult. Some are just Skeptics. Skeptics makeup 60% of the population and seek only evidence. They believe it, but getting this evidence can be difficult.

Bramber reads

If the clairvoyance feels good in the session and you are fighting on the go, that person is not happy. It is the type of person who is usually not pleased about anything, and the reader "knows" this before starting and can generally be adjusted. In such situations, the visionary must look to "intuition."

From time to time, you may need to choke to let go of the person. But you know you did a great job. I don't think it's great to read when others agree. It's frustrating and doesn't allow you to affect your skills or get stuck in holes you can't get out of it. It may be annoying to you, but they are getting in the way. It's up to you to get the information in full and do something with it. You started by forwarding the message, and you must expect it without seeing it yourself. Objects may retain later, depending on the conclusion. Mental Amnesia and some people don't recognize certain things in the session but keep them to themselves. So, don't guess! Always do it with your intuition. That's not a mistake! Whatever someone else says.

Free Will - Couldn't Have Said It Better Myself!

A story of a psychic friend and some excellent advice I 100% agree with:

"One of the best compliments I've ever had was that I told why a psychiatrist took seven years to contact her 20 minutes after the session began," I said, I told him about the client, but I gave her another perspective. She refused his solution because of her free will. If, after receiving possible events, when to expect them and how to handle them when they occur, she agreed if she feels better than in recent years. It was A few months later. She called again to thank life for her continued changes and improvements, telling her she was the one who made these changes, not me. I point out the possibilities and think about them. It was possible. She is more satisfied with her life now than for a long time. Scammers can't have this effect, but good clairvoyance can hold it for life. It requires "extraordinary insights." Nor does it mean that every reading changes the subject and your life. A person in need of help must get it physically and mentally. A reputable and reliable clairvoyant is happy to contact your doctor if you determine that your doctor needs you, or if your tests free you from both conditions. It should not involve you in this business without thinking. Jumping into an unprepared psychic field is as dangerous as trying to climb Everest without equipment or practice. If you are interested, please go slowly-the study. Sitters/customers can turn around to avoid certain events. There is almost nothing inevitable in life. The decisions we make determine the activities that take place. These events are expected and subject to change. The greatest gift we have is free will and choice in our lives. Never give up."

BEE

Bees can fly. But Bee doesn't know; they can't fly. Or can you do it? According to scientific research (as you may have heard), bees must not run. Their wings are too small for the body, making flight impossible. But they do it because they "don't know" they can't run. They fly because they have no restrictions. If you know, you can't do it, find out what you can't do. A determined person can prove that this person is wrong and can do it. But you can see that others are doing the same. We discern throughout our lives that we cannot do it. The perspective is not unrealistic! Extending our consciousness is a new sensation, six sensations (or ESP or psychological skills). Moderate skills come from one part of the brain, and other gifts come from another part of the brain. In either case, we do not know the exact science of the problem. I know the problem exists and is working. It's a reality, and we can do it. Don't limit yourself. Do not listen to anyone who tries to restrict your knowledge. It is possible, and you can do it. Time, practice and patience are essential. But it's happening, so don't forget to expect it to happen. Faster than I expected! If you think it happens. So, you are afraid to approach. Don't be scared, just think positively and see the happy ending.

Universe's Role

The universe plays the most critical role. The spiritual information we receive focuses on what is happening by predicting what is happening in the future, or what we will see and who we will be. It is coming to us what happens through their thoughts. I think you have read all the above. I feel like I'm absorbing energy at that point. However, the reading may change in the next two moments. There are two kinds of people, one is changing their thoughts or attitudes, and others discern the prediction is changing their will.

The universe shows that you are on the right path-I.E. Deja Vu, coincidence, and so on. DejaVu-I believes there are many reasons. I will tell you why through my reading and beliefs. We were dreaming of this or more events recently or recently when Deja Vu happened. It is a theory. The main reason

Deja Vu occurs is that it creates a draft of life before it enters life. During this process, we make decisions and challenges. And in our lives, we choose a path. But before we get into this life, see how it works, what events happen, how they happen, and what happens when you choose a choice or route Let's look. Let's look at different scenarios and see what we want to do. It is called a scan. It's a bit like TV, but more realistic. A scan is a name Sylvia Brown uses in this book in this process. We don't remember this for a lifetime, but I think "Deja Vu" happened before. It happened before-at least during the scan. You have scanned events, and some of your souls "remember" those events.

There is always a reason for an opportunity. It's not a coincidence. These also inform you that you are on the right path in life. The universe is each one of us. We are the universe, and the universe is the United

States. The world is all made up of objects, plants, people, places, etc. We are all made up of our thoughts. Our experience came from pure thought and fear. So, it's easy to say, think positively! When you become positive, this cheery wave returns to you! The universe seems to react to the waves. If you do negative things, you will eventually get back to the score. What you do will come back to you. You are doing something positive. It will come back to you.

Some Homework

Test the universe now! You can check it out, and it will answer! I've read other books and love these examples, so give flowers a try. I like purple, so I chose purple. So, I asked to bring purple flowers into the universe (in my eyes, energy increases if it helps you). Don't hesitate to make them bigger. It is in many formats. You can see not only real flowers but also photos of flowers and hear clues about the story. Purple is the favorite color of those who send flowers to Narrator history. There was a request from space, a purple flower. Of course, mentioning purple flowers is not enough. So, I republished this idea (more on this time) and asked for a real purple flower. I must have given this idea many times!

If you use energy there for something and are not afraid of this idea (since it just won't come in), this will happen. You must think about it, and you know it, and it happens. Again, the only problem is what you think is happening and whether it should happen. I believe there are all reasons. You can find the universe and know this knowledge about energy, and in this way, you can do it better for you. Don't try to rethink it!

Seven Major Chakras

Crown Chakra: Dark Purple-Connect with the Heart. It also controls the upper brain (cerebrum), cerebral cortex, and central nervous system. An imbalance of infection types can lead to headaches, sinuses, neuralgia, and ear problems—third Eye Charka (Forehead).

Dark Purple Indigo: It's named because the Third Eye is here. It is our supernatural power. It also refers to the lower brain (cerebellar) and the central nervous system.

Heart Chakra Green: It is our ability to love ourselves and others. It Performs the heart, thymus, and circulation. Respiratory infections can cause asthma, allergies, and even heart problems.

Solar Plexus Chakra: This is our strength. This chakra becomes unbalanced when you strengthen someone or something. It controls the sympathetic nervous system, digestion, and metabolism. You may have a problem with your breast, lungs, pancreas, spleen, stomach, liver, adrenal glands, or kidneys.

Sacral Plexus Chakra: Orange-Our wish is in this chakra. This chakra reveals all kinds of desires and needs. Problems can occur if there is a problem with the imbalance of the lower abdomen, intestines, ovaries, uterine prostate, or genitals.

Root or base chakra: Red security (that is, finance, etc.) is the main attribute of this chakra. It guides the adrenal glands, kidneys, spine, and colon. Unbalanced kidney problems can cause hip and groin problems and imbalances. I also noticed low back pain while working on this chakra imbalance problem.

Aura: The aura is a continually changing, beautifully colored energy field that surrounds all living things. It's like an oval egg that surrounds our body. The atmosphere is made up of many layers, starting with the innermost layer closest to the collection and ending approximately 4-5 feet from the body. The upper layer is another part of a person's consciousness, where the inner layer is connected to the body, followed by the upper layers, including the emotional layer, the metal layer, and the metal layer. Our aura comes from conscious and unconscious thoughts, feelings, and the energy that flows through our bodies. Your health is affected by the condition of your atmosphere. Aura treatments are an essential part of Reiki sessions.

Chakras: Chakras are subtle energy converters. You always receive the universal life energy that surrounds us and translates it into the different frequencies that our creative energy system requires to maintain our health. There are seven critical chakras: root, sacrum, solar plexus, heart, neck, third eye, and crown. The root chakra (lowest) provides the low frequencies needed for physical survival, and the highest or crown chakra provides the mental energy level. Each chakra corresponds to a layer of the aura. Chaka can reduce the amount of sensitive energy and accumulate negative emotions and thoughts that affect your health. Chakra treatment is an integral part of Reiki treatment.

Meridians: Meridians are the way subtle energy flows through your body. Meridians contain energy points, commonly called acupuncture points or shiatsu points. Each meridian is usually connected to an organ or physical system of the body to provide subtle life energy. As you can see from the chakra table alone, not only all chakras but also the balance between the aura and the meridian is essential. It is so complicated that we can't go into the meridian anymore. The above explanation is enough to understand why an aura/chakra balance is essential.

Exercise

Contact Spirit Guide

Our expectations for how Spirit contact us are often too high. The existence of the mind is as thinking energy. Therefore, it makes sense to contact us about our thoughts. But how can you tell the difference? Ideas sound like their own and can be more explicit and structured and eloquent. My tip is if you have a question, and the answer comes before the article is complete! If you can calm down like meditation, you may be able to recognize these thoughts better. It also applies to the recognition of spirits that speak to you and your spirit guide! Ask questions, and see how you feel. You can take the time to seek advice if needed. The answer is usually available to you. That is why they are here. Sometimes we must be patient, a lesson. Spirits / Universes work with you, but not you. They know what we don't know, they know our goal, and perhaps we don't. They often await us to get rid of doubts, blockages, and other distractions that can undermine the work they are trying to teach.

If you feel or see someone in the distance through meditation (or a dream), this is often a new guide waiting to join you and expect to be ready. It can be a leader who has been with you for 40 years, not only through you (through your spiritual reading and centrality if you choose these paths) but also through you. The guide that has been waiting for you since your birth. Won't you wait for such a guide and be patient? You don't like it, but it's an example of how you can change your thoughts, expectations, and patience. Everything happens in your own time. Everything happens for a reason.

A psychometric measurement is the explanation of every living being by an aura or energy field. The atmosphere is continually changing and moving, but everything about this person, this animal, the plant is in them from birth to the present-everything they experience, think, and feel. Ready to develop everything. It is also important to remember that personal energy can also bring into being. Stick to everything that touches her.

You can also import it into a photo. To find something about someone (including animals), you can first keep something that belongs to that person. It can be clothes, carpets, photos (collars, hair, etc.). It's a psychological measure. Get a pen and paper and write down what you think. Press and hold an item to open it and accept it to see what happens. Make sure you get results right away.

The longer you sit and think, the more hinder your thinking. Just stop and don't disturb your beliefs and expectations. Think about it right away? Do you think it smells, or do you see anything in your mind? If it makes no sense, write it down. What you are doing is "releasing" their energy full of information, and while you do this, you can connect with people and suddenly receive messages from them. You don't have to be present for telepathy to work!

Mental (Energy) Vampire

Remember that you must always immerse yourself in the light of the white universe and seek protection from your guides and angels. However, even with this protection, you will encounter a mental / energy vampire. You're doing it, and you just don't know.

There are many types and levels of psychic vampires. There are human spiritual vampires and other spiritual vampires in the world. All you need to know was when this happened to you and how you can protect yourself and others! A psychic vampire is a person/entity that draws energy directly from you, deprives you of power, and, if you continue this low-energy pattern, does so. You need to get rid of it and increase your protection and aura to keep these people away. Many human spiritual vampires are unaware of doing this to others. They are unaware of the negativity they use and the use of other energies.

These spiritual vampires can be very dangerous, and this is a serious business. You can get energy directly from you until you are no longer alive (in this respect). You need to learn to recognize the signs to protect yourself. We strongly recommend that you take precautions to protect yourself before a dangerous situation occurs. The body has apparent features that are perceived, but it also recognizes the underlying emotions of intuition when you cannot see the obvious. The obvious is people who always live with negative emotions! Jealousy of pessimism and hatred, envy, anger, resentment, and darkness, consumed like suspect, disbelief, despair, fear, and always perceiving the dark side of life! When these negative emotions are there, they are already ruining your energy. You must protect yourself from it. People with these negative feelings (and so on) attract lower points. Its constant negativity of emotions attracts astral presence at low levels. They also act as a negative energy/thought that causes negativity. It is a wave effect. Everyone within range feels the impact of the waves. Be careful not to get in the way. Darkness is also attracted to light. Also, if you are just trying to improve your mental skills, you will be more vulnerable to energy vampires. Because you are not always protecting yourself and practicing to "know" about such things.

Protection

My first idea is to remind everyone that visualization is enormous. Imagine what you can do to block what you don't want to receive, and when you don't want to. I immediately asked to stand in the white light, even in the mirror containing the white light. In this way, you can "see" what they are doing, even if that person's subconsciousness is half that size. I do not know that a spiritual vampire is an energy vampire. If you have too much energy or feel uncomfortable, focus on a remote location or another location.

Energy goes where attention flows. Performance can be positive or negative. It is how we learn to put themselves in this life and how to work. Sometimes it's best to turn your back instead of "paying attention" (paying energy).

Anonymous Description of Energy Flow

When the white light is in you-when you merge with the white light-the emotions that come out of you are what you feel in that light (it is peaceful, fearless, any form of love but not)—feeling of neutrality and "carelessness" (backup and charging). It is different from what you would think if the light was only "around you." At this point, you feel the need for fear and protection and security.

Energy goes where attention flows, and when we are in the light, source, and spirit of God, no matter what we do, our "hopes" always come true. Everyone who thinks about us is in the light we "feel" (we must be afraid of whether we know empathy or not. When we feel this energy, we understand. It's someone who exudes fear or something.

And if you choose to pray for someone who feels unappealing or personal, we move this light of love. We lose love because we feel loved, taken care of, and comforted, and they are ours. It is an emotion that spreads to all "personal" people. We do this, give them the opportunity to move, connect, and push themselves to the same warm light or spirit source. When they are ready and otherwise (until ready), they leave. We start reading, listening, and learning about everything, and our network of people experience, know, and "feel" this networking. We experience this network through mutual empathy.

For Energy Cleaners: Ask the universe to surround you and your subject again with white light. Instead of stealing energy, look at it in the white light of UNIVERSES. If so, you have their powers sucked, there are some holes in the aura they need to fix, and their problem is that they too are energy suckers. You can openly and openly tell them what you know to make up for the negativity they compromise. They must improve their situation and either get rid of it or put up with it and stop seeing it as a problem. There are three options: change, resign, reduce the irony of the problem (change the perspective of the situation), or get out of the situation completely. If you continue to feel this way, you should do everything possible to stay away from them. You can't allow them to suck your energy.

Smear

Lubrication is the most common and most recommended process when you need to clean a negative in your home (for example, previous discussions or mood-dependent emotions). There are many reasons to smear, but I don't think it will spread. There is no adverse effect. Simply put, Sage frees your home from negativity. White sage is said to be the best, but all are effective. You can point to yourself, your family, your car, any object, and so on. Some say that you regularly ruin your home, much like cleaning your home every week or every other week. And some say that monthly practice is good. Do what you think is right. When talking to your house, focus on the front and rear door frames. Walk around every room and focus on every corner. If it is possible, to try painting outside the house, on the property, on the windows and doors.

Incense Protection

If you need to get rid of the negativity around you, I highly recommend it. It comes with excellent cleaning. Sand Bake 3 Sandalwood incense once a day for seven days. (If you still need it after seven days, burn three sticks once a week.) After applying the incense stick, say three times a day as follows.

"Because this incense burns out,

Today, all enemies vitiated.

I am no longer worried.

I cannot do anything.

Immunize me forever.

And it looks like my will! "

Input

Be mentally aware and open and be more aware of your skills. The more conscious you are, the more sensitive you are to your surroundings and the various energy fields around you. When doing this, you must interpret the energy through a lot of practice and diligence. The main thing I always say to others is that you must meditate. This word has many symbolic meanings, but it is not the one you are likely to hear. All you must do is sit still and look inside. There are many ways to meditate.

When you are asleep, you can accept messages from other spirits, leaders, and the universe. The state from sleep to waking up is called the alpha state achieved in meditation. Not only does meditation help accept messages, but it also adapts to intuition in reflection and daily life to receive instructions about notes and common questions. You may or may not need a piece because you don't know how quiet or noisy your home or environment is. Choose the one you find most useful. Relax without sleeping! Some people want to meditate on a sound machine that makes the sounds of the sea and rain. At this point, it's entirely up to you.

For many, it is challenging to think nothing during meditation. We meditate on many thoughts that pass through my head. Finally (unless you worry) you can push in only one idea (whether worried or boring). Another thought came in, and you can take it further. The Master of Buddhism gave another idea when it was more challenging to think when meditating; he said, "clear heart" when inhaling and "don't know when exhaling." Change the vocals to your liking.

CHAPTER 6: ESSENTIAL MEDITATION AND AFFIRMATION

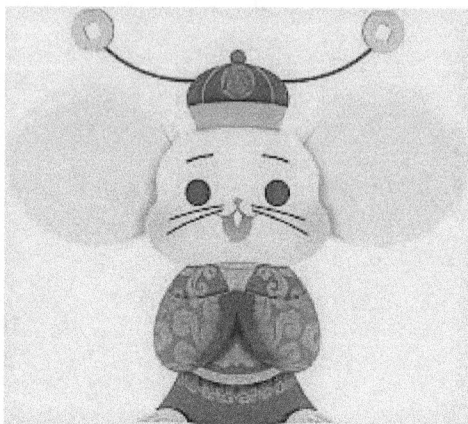

Meditation is the discipline that purifies the mind and seeks your inner self. In the state of meditation, the external world is almost entirely closed, and the subconscious retains sensory inputs. What you achieve is not only a way of controlling yourself but open to all other types of psychological impressions. People who meditate regularly have high energy levels, low blood pressure, and little stress. This condition makes your account better, so a focused mind can perform tasks more efficiently.

During meditation, your brain activity falls from beta (daily; widely awake) to alpha (sleep, sleepy, or relaxed). So, the trick is to go there. There are many ways to do this, but there are several. Everything should put upon for personal work. Relieve stress or raise awareness. When doing mental training, start at the end of meditation.

Health That Relieves Stress and Builds Confidence

Health is a positive concept, as advocated by over 190 signatories of the World Health Organization. The WHO definition of health means that mental health cannot bring off by the prevention or treatment of disorders alone. It must address a broader range of issues affecting the mental health of every part of society. Mental health refers to various activities directly or indirectly related to the elements of psychological well-being within the WHO definition of health. It is associated with promoting welfare, preventing mental disorders, and treating and rehabilitating those affected by mental disorders.

Mental health is an essential part of an individual's overall health. All thought processes carried out in mind, so ideas are born in mind, and all kinds of directions that guide, shape, and regulate communication, actions, and behaviors and determine personal and social aspects carry out from the heart—function and adaptation.

Health depends on your physical and mental condition. Health usually means well-being or freedom from disease. Thus, mental health can refer to a healthy mental state or state of liberation from mental health or mental illness. The mind and bodywork simultaneously in harmony. A healthy body requires a healthy account, and a healthy mind has a healthy sense, so proper analysis of the body and mind is necessary to understand personality. Mental health is a complete and harmonious function of the whole nature.

If it accredits that mental health is not just a lack of mental illness, then the positive aspects of mental health are underlined. Health is a positive state of well-being, not just an absence of disease. People in emotional, physical, and social welfare fulfill their responsibilities in their lives, function effectively in their daily lives, and are content with themselves and their interpersonal relationships.

Positive psychology, psychological well-being, quality of life, and well-being are used as synonyms for mental health. Happiness is undoubtedly the desired goal of human beings, and we are all striving to achieve it. Happiness refers to the harmonious functioning of a person's physical and psychological aspects as a subjective sensation, joy, and satisfaction. Happiness is a composite measure of physical/biological, psychological/mental, and social well-being. Biological indicators of well-being include health status, health consciousness, use of health habits, and behavior in maintaining health. Psychosocial indicators of well-being include mental health, cognitive function, positive emotions, adjustment, and satisfaction with life experience, comfort.

Information technology has transformed the world into a global village (McLuhan, 1969). People's attitudes and behaviors seem like a significant departure from past communities. The values of consumption, individualism, materialism, hedonism, sadism, and masochism have increased significantly, and the susceptibility of others to suffering has decreased substantially (Bhargava and Raina, 2007). All types of anxiety, physical, mental, and social can affect people's minds, causing anxiety, frustration, stress, tension, mismatches, personal and social problems. It all involves a person's mental health.

Therefore, good mental health is essential to achieve and enjoy full health. Good mental health ensures the emergence of healthy ideas and tools that control personal and social functioning and adaptation.

Definition of Mental Health

Mental health delineates as:

"Mental health means the ability of an individual to build a harmonious relationship with others, to participate in and contribute to changes in the social and physical environment. Utilizing the ability to achieve the smooth and balanced satisfaction of an inconsistent proprietary drive.

In 1995, Allport dealt with a healthy personality and prescribed tests for normal and mature adults instead of neurosis. He pointed out that healthy people were not subject to unconscious conflicts, but adults with obsessions had these conflicts. Mental health is a mental state characterized by mental peace, harmony, and content. It relates to a person's lack of both mental and physical disability and debilitating symptoms.

According to Maslow (1970), those who have exhausted their potential lead us to the formation of "positive psychology" and free us from a negative approach. He always studied to find the healthiest and most mature aspects of human nature. Sortorives (1983) states that "mental health is the equilibrium between an individual and the world around him, the harmony between himself and others, and the coexistence of the reality and environment of himself and others."

In 1992, Kumar warned not to confuse mental health with mental illness. That mental health can serve as an indicator of how well a person was able to meet their social, emotional, and physical environmental needs. If he/she is in a situation where he/she does not have the proper strategy to handle it effectively, he/she will be mentally stressed. This mental stress reflects symptoms such as anxiety, tension, restlessness, and despair. If a person feels it too long and too healthy, then these symptoms can manifest themselves (or become a "syndrome") and represent a disease. According to Kumar, mental health is the study of a person's mental state before they get sick.

According to Park (1995), "mental health is a well-balanced development of an individual's personality and emotional attitude that enables us to live in harmony with others." Singh (2000) defined mental health as the ability to love.

Mental health can descend from their behavior. A person's behavior can be seen and interpreted by others, depending on their values and beliefs. Thus, mental health is a state of emotional, psychological, and social well-being, characterized by interpersonal satisfaction, productive behavior, and coping positive self-image, and emotional stability.

Mental health is a component of overall health that includes interrelated physical, mental, emotional, social, and cultural health. Bhargava and Aurora (2006) point out that psychological well-being produces the health and excellence of all human health. Therefore, good physical or mental health requires general psychological health, as it relates to the reality and skills of people and workers to deal with problems and challenges.

Bhargava refers to mental health as the right and balanced development of intelligence, creativity, reasoning, emotions, mindfulness, and initiative, a social aspect that faces daily problems and diverse challenges without losing patience. Various factors play an essential role in shaping a sane person. These include personal resources, social support, integrated private structure, individual quality of life, pleasant family atmosphere, a good understanding of the community, cultural and religious harmony.

Tripathi et al. (2006) pointed out the perceptions of India that can make a positive contribution to the state of mental health in modern life. Ego Absence, Sthitapragya, and the Anasakti States, Maitra, Karuna, and Mudita. The perceptions have given in the classical Indian text complement and complement our holistic view of mental health.

However, mental health is an excellent ability to live and enjoy a good life. An investigation of internal psychological states and processes, or Chittavritti, is one of the central themes of classical Indian text. Indian thought seeks to understand and analyze natural tendencies, desires, passions, etc. to control them consciously. The purpose of this control is to deal with negative emotions and values such as Trishna, Raga, Dwesh and eliminate them, and replace them with positive emotions and benefits such as love and compassion. It is to enhance and refine personality.

Based on the above discussion, mental health can explain the state of well-being in which an individual can recognize their abilities, cope with the stresses of ordinary life, be productive and fruitful, and contribute to their community.

Thus, a person's mental health is a dynamic or continuously changing state. Several components interact with each other. Enough sense of security, self-esteem, contact with reality, genuine physical desire and ability to satisfy them, self-knowledge, increased self-confidence, warm relationships with others, emotional security, unity of life philosophy, neighbors Ability to take responsibility for others and fellow humans, orientation. The growth and maximization of your potential, the ability to deal with and influence the environment with competence, knowledge, and creativity, the overall acceptance of yourself and others, spontaneity, the freshness of creativity and vision, and healthy Sense of humor, strong reaction, ability to understand problems, ability to make decisions, solution-oriented attitude, positive thinking, awareness, ability to maximize one's potential, emotional development, creativity, intelligence and spirituality, The ability to face and react to problems without losing patience, strengths and lessons for the future, the ability to analyze an expanded self, the ability to be accurate.

Some authors describe some indicators of good mental health.

According to Maslow and Mitelman (1951), the following are normal mental health:

1. Enough security

2. Appropriate self-assessment

3. Appropriate spontaneity and emotionality

4. Efficient contact with reality

5. Relevant physical needs and the ability to satisfy them

6. Proper self-awareness

7. Personality integration and consistency

8. Appropriate goals in life

9. Ability to learn from experience

10. Ability to meet group requirements

11. Enough liberation from cultural groups

Schultz (1977) examined the following seven criteria for mental health.

1. Increased confidence

2. The warm relationship between self and others

3. emotional safety

4. realistic perception

5. Skills and tasks

6. Self-purpose

7. Standardization of life philosophy

Compared to the numerous criteria proposed by Maslow, Kittleman, and Schultz, Park, and Park (1977) described only three significant features:

1. You feel good, safe, and appropriate, accept your benefits and limitations, and have self-esteem and confidence.

2. You think right about others, so you can develop friendships and loving behaviors, and build trust in others. Therefore, a person can take responsibility for his / her neighbors and fellow humans.

3. A sane person can meet the demands of life. He/she does something about the problems that arise. He/she sets reasonable goals, takes daily responsibilities, thinks about himself, and makes decisions himself. He/she does not cry through his feelings of "fear, anger, love, and guilt."

Johnson (1997) has shown that a person's mental health is either dynamic or continuously changing:

1. The person is autonomous and independent and can work or interdependent with others. He/she can also consider the decisions and actions of others but cannot by others.

2. The person concentrates on the growth and maximizes its potential.

3. One can withstand the uncertainties of life with hope and a positive outlook without the

knowledge of the future, facing the challenges of everyday life.

4. The person must be self-respecting and realistically aware of their abilities and limitations.

5. A person can deal with and influence the environment in a competent and creative way.

6. People are realistic and need to act accordingly.

7. Deal with crises from family and friends because the person can cope with stress, can withstand the pressure of life and feelings of fear and grief, and know that stress does not last forever. You can get support for it.

An Indian view of mental health can comprehend the reason by Bhatnagar (2000) and Singh (2002). Some of the

critical indicators proposed by Bhatnagar are:

1. Accepting yourself and others.

2. Spontaneity, creativity, the freshness of vision, healthy sense of humor.

3. The typical reaction, ability to understand problems, decision-making ability, and solution-oriented attitude.

4. Individual autonomy, credibility, and responsibility for yourself.

5. Healthy interpersonal relationships, adaptability, and quality of life.

6. Positive thinking, awareness, and maximizing your potential.

7. Emotional maturity, sensitivity, empathy, ability to manage emotions effectively.

8. Achieve your peace and harmonize with others.

9. The ability to make creative and constructive contributions to bring about desirable changes in the physical environment and socio-cultural context.

Singh (2002) found a mentally healthy person with the following characteristics:

1. Development of emotion, creativity, intelligence, and spirituality.

2. Maintain a mutually rewarding social relationship.

3. Ability to cope with problems and issues without losing patience, capacity to respond to enough power, and learn lessons for the future.

4. Have confidence, assertion, sensitivity, and empathy for the suffering of others.

5. Constructively prepare for the fun use of loneliness, participate in fun and games.

6. Laugh in enjoyable, fun, fantastic, and incredible situations.

Bhargava (2002) show some indicators of good mental health:

1. Full acceptance of yourself and others.

2. You need the ability to analyze your expanded self. They must be aware of their benefits, accept limitations, feel comfortable and peaceful to themselves, set themselves reasonable goals, and can make their own decisions.

3. The person should have the ability to manage himself by analyzing self-concept and self-realization.

4. As a member of society, we need to understand social responsibility and build

healthy interpersonal relationships that are in harmony with other methods to solve community-wide problems.

5. You should prepare your life plan considering your skills and abilities and be very systematic with a realistic view of the environment.

6. You should be able to meet life's demands and take on daily responsibility.

7. You should be able to understand the problems at every stage of your life and adapt to try to solve them in this situation.

8. To bring the environment to life, in social and cultural conditions, we need to contribute to creative and constructive ways to bring about desirable changes in the physical environment.

9. You should have a clear vision in all areas of life and think positively and innovatively to make swift decisions.

10. You need to be radical, flexible, and accessible to adapt to your requirements and time.

11. One must pay attention to the existence of the Almighty, or "Ishwar," and all actions or ideas should be devoted to the power of the Almighty in the world, and in no way meaningful. It gives peace and happiness throughout life.

12. To manage emotions effectively so that an emotionally balanced person feels emotionally safe, you need to develop humor, joy, and enthusiasm.

13. If you want to keep real-world requirements in violation of shared values and norms, you need to adapt. There are also three things to consider when making a step: time, place, and person.

14. We need the ability to distinguish good from evil. The person should be able to ignore

fears of unknown or speculative thinking and control fears of better mental health.

15. You should consistently develop your integrated personality.

16. At a minimum, you should set a satisfactory level according to all the realities of your life. Otherwise, you will not feel the satisfaction of life. Instead of criticizing others, you need to evaluate and overcome your weaknesses.

Factors That Affect Mental Health

Personality structures, relatives, castes, classes, friends, districts, neighborhoods, labor organizations, clubs, groups, communities, cultures, religions, etc., play an essential role in shaping a person's mental health. Pradan et al. (2006) divided them into six factors that affect a person's mental health.

1. Individual factors include the biological structure of the individual. It harmonizes with one's life, vitality, finding meaning in life, emotional resilience and strength, spirituality, and positive identity.

2. Factors of interpersonal relationships include effective communication, helping others, intimacy, and separation and connection (attribution), maintaining a balance between family and social support.

3. Socio-cultural factors include a sense of communication, access to appropriate resources, intolerance of violence, social organization, time orientation, and environmental control.

4. Self-esteem plays an essential role in mental health decisions. People with high self-esteem have less stress and tension and are much more responsible.

5. The internal control site is related to mental health.

6. Emotional intelligence, in terms of general components such as public health, healthy coping style, empathy, happiness, apathy, neurosis, stressful events, and mood swings.

Causes and Prevalence of Ill Mental Health

The growth and development of children are not as smooth and continuous as children would like, due to the various disadvantages affecting children at home, school, and society. Children may be born with specific disabilities or develop social, psychological, or physiological problems. It can ultimately affect the development of their abilities and prevent him from working as he should or cause him to have adverse reactions to other people or society. It can also lead to children with disabilities and learning difficulties.

A study by (Lapouse and Monk, 1958, 1964) showed that the prevalence of behavioral deviations in school-age children decreased with age. Infants aged 6-8 were far more biased in behavior than older infants (9-12). Boys performed better than girls. The frequency of behavioral deviations is higher in black and white children. There seemed to be little difference in the rate of behavioral differences between the siblings alone. Banik (1972) mentioned the incidence of appropriate behavior in elementary school.

Two categories-behavioral issues and personality issues exist over here. In the first category, 10.3% of children (more boys than girls) were aggressive, 10.5% hated school, 6.7% were wary, and 8.4% were restless. In the second category, 11.5% lacked confidence, and 10.6% required concentration. Loneliness, irritability, and stuttering are present in nearly 7% of children.

In 1969, Muralidharan reported that a smaller family system promotes the development of problem behaviors in children. Almost all studies indicate a high prevalence of problem behaviors in boys, especially behavioral disorders. No disturbing action occurs in a vacuum. Behavioral disorders are terms assigned according to cultural rules rather than "things" that lie outside the social context (Burbach, 1981). (Kasinath, 2003) observe that mental health plays a vital role in expressing student personality traits. He also reported that students with good mental health performed well in all school subjects. External control sites are significantly associated with psychological adjustment problems. Studies have shown a positive contribution of social support to mental well-being.

How Can A Psychologist Help?

Psychologists can evaluate the extent to which each school promotes mental health and assists people and students with disabilities, including teachers and other staff. All schools should have an overall mental health treatment plan that includes:

1. A holistic school approach to promote mental health for all children.

2. Active support for teachers to support children who are distracted or withdrawn.

3. Non-stigmatic and available support for students and staff who are not only accessible but have problems is useable.

4. Active connection to parents, psychiatric services for children and adolescents, and other related services.

5. Manage all transitions to and from school to minimize associated mental health issues,

including unusual changes such as exclusions.

6. Like many aspects of the exam, it should reduce teacher stress rather than increase it.

Roles of parents and professionals in promoting mental health

We are as responsible for our emotional health as we are for our physical health. It's up to us to access support and what kind of support we use to help us manage our emotions and behaviors. Parents and professionals can play an essential role in promoting the mental health of children. Such support begins with the basics of maintaining boundaries and follows the knowledge of how to communicate effectively.

I. Observe Limits: Parents and professionals can help promote positive mental health among young people by merely teaching the appropriate rules and limits and the risk of injury.

II. Power of communication: You can convey all your feelings through actions and body language without having to tell or express your feelings to anyone. 54% of all communications are nonverbal, and only 7% is verbal. When we say something, we can communicate what we feel-the the tone we use when speaking can convey the way we feel. It may not always be "angry" or "exciting," but anger and excitement are in our way of speaking. Body language, behavior, voice tones, what someone says or doesn't say is what psychiatric professionals, most therapists, and counselors listen to and pay attention to how they do it.

Use Total communication

Children and adolescents may find it challenging to convey their feelings to others. Sometimes you don't have the right words, or you can't express yourself verbally. As a result, some therapists use art, theatre, drama, and music when working with young people. However, parents and professionals can see what young people are telling about their body language and behavior and hear the tone of their voice to determine how they feel at a time.

III. Emotional Ability-Understanding why you think that way can help you learn how to deal with your daily life. Young people know their feelings well, but they don't always fully understand why they feel that way. It makes it difficult for young people to deal with certain situations and when they do occur.

IV. Ask a Question-Once you know precisely what a young person is feeling, you can take the next step and ask a question to ask what he felt. However, doing so is also an art. Asking "closed" items that can be answered "yes" or "no" is far less useful than asking "open" questions that encourage people to give more detailed answers.

V. Searching for Options or Advice-Being unsure what to do in a situation, young people may seek advice from others on a specific issue. Young people often think that adults are "experts" in the life problems they have Correct. How else can young people get information about difficulties or find ways to deal with them? Maybe you don't know the options available to you to solve or deal with a situation. Therefore, exploring alternatives can be a useful strategy.

VI. Practice constructive criticism-Critical and rarely praised young people often have low self-esteem and confidence. Therefore, constructive criticism is essential to help young people realize what they are doing well and what they are not doing. Constructive criticism is saying what a person is doing, letting them know what "good" is, and then saying what they are doing "bad."

Adolescent Mental Health

People experience the most difficult changes in young ones. There are dramatic changes in physique and cognitive ability. Adolescence marks the beginning of sexuality, but mental skills lead to the sophistication needed to apply mathematical formulas and use tricky words and sentences. Between the ages of 12 and 18, changes in body shape, development of secondary sexual characteristics, hormonal and biochemical alterations form the basis of mature sexual function. Due to the changes they are experiencing, and adolescents are beginning to revise their views on themselves. Social relationships outside the family are becoming increasingly important. It is not uncommon to rebel against the authority of parents during adolescence. Strange but true, adolescence is generally regarded as the most challenging period of adolescent youth restlessly looking for its identity.

Havighurst (1973) points out some of the youth development tasks:

1. Build new and more mature relationships with your bisexual mates.

2. Achieve male or female social roles.

3. Accept your body and use it effectively.

4. Achieve emotional independence from parents and other adults.

5. Preparation for marriage and family life.

6. Preparing for an economic career.

7. Acquisition of values and ethical system as action guidelines-Development of ideology.

8. Hope and achieve socially responsible behavior.

All this makes adolescence an era of emotional confusion, dark reflection, high drama, and heightened sensitivity. It's time for rebellion and behavior experiments. It's not wondered that adolescent mental health is gaining a lot of attention as adolescents become more aware of the unfortunate consequences of reduced mental health.

Taking on new responsibilities and roles that can pose risks, renegotiate relationships with adults and peers in families and communities, try things that are symbolic of adult life, and ask questions is about youth development. The natural part of life that sets the rules of social customs.

It is a severe stage in life, and existing mental health problems can intensify. Habits may escalate, sleep may be disturbed, and eating habits may be overly generous or restricted. In girls, hormonal fluctuations often cause irregular emotions. Many adolescents practice a variety of behaviors that are not characteristic of their usual selves. Under these circumstances, mental health disorders prevent an adolescent from fulfilling his physical, psychological, and social potential if left untreated.

Anxiety increasingly suppresses adolescent psychosocial development, persistent self-interrogation that impairs self-confidence, and can interfere with the development of decision-making skills. Failure to handle intense emotions soundly can lead to adolescents expressing pain and numbness through violence, self-harm, isolation, reckless behavior, and the use of alcohol and illegal drugs (Sandhu, 2006).

The Need for School-Based Intervention Planning

Many studies have shown that relevant factors such as school environment and attitudes of teachers, classmates on teaching methods, and overall equipment available in the classroom or school adversely affect the mental health status of children.

The expectations of parents, legal guardians, and teachers play a significant role in increasing pressure on young children. In addition to letting children score and grade in school and college, most parents want their children to be wise, intelligent, and successful in all competitions. Worse, in some cases, parents want their children to achieve dreams they (parents) could not make. Teachers also expect their students to have excellent academic and extracurricular activities. If a child does not live up to their expectations, they will not only be disappointed but will take care of themselves.

Young people spend a lot of time at school, providing a meaningful social context. The school becomes a social lab for them because they make friends here. Here they go into constructive or destructive action. Here they understand the agreement/disagreement between their inner desires and determinations (Sharma and Srivastava, 2006).

Adolescents are confused by the fact that the school rejects almost everything they think. Young people demand freedom, school values , and discipline. Young people strive for identity, autonomy, and connection, but school experience counteracts natural desires and is a hallmark of this developmental stage. An inflexible curriculum and schedule keep young people in the same cultural and intellectual form, overlooking a diversity of talents and opportunities. They emphasize the development of abstract knowledge at the expense of imagination, communication skills, leadership, aesthetics, or manual skills to show the dignity of work. Schools are trying to make them virtual robots, all of which are handled by similar courses, teaching materials, instructions, and assessment techniques (Sharma and Srivastava, 2006).

Under these circumstances, parents and teachers need to build a warm and trusting relationship with young people. It will increase the student's connection to the classroom and allow them to discuss any issues they may encounter. The importance of a flexible school environment cannot accent, but this is, of course, a significant challenge.

"Children's mental health gives us an idea of the next generation of adult mental health. Children and adolescent psychiatric services are part of the responsibility of health and the local government. Still, children and adolescent mental health the consequences of inadequate attention to health are the ongoing suffering of children and their families, as well as constant spiral child abuse: delinquency in boys over the age of 34, family breakdown, and adult mental illness.

It can cause mental health problems in children and adolescents. "Regular school and university physical exams for emotional, behavioral, and school-related issues, as well as regular physical exams, are for teachers and parents to have anxiety disorders, habit disorders, attention deficit hyperactivity disorder in their children. It helps to recognize problems such as early and take countermeasures. Early detection and proper management of these problems not only improve the life of the child but also help parents deal with their child's restrictions.

Issues related to positive mental health have become increasingly important in recent years. Good psychological well-being does not merely mean that there is no mental health problem, but emotional creativity, the development of intelligence and spirituality, initiatives, questions, and lessons for the future. They are developing and maintaining social relationships for learning, self-expression, and empathy (Surender, 2002).

Attitude

Humans are indeed all living things and adjust throughout their lives. Most of the changes we make aren't important enough and even don't get registered in our heads to make them look like reflex actions. Little be relevant to such adjustments. To include a learning program, take on a job, work on a project outside your home country, get married, or look for a separation or divorce, you need to adjust to varying degrees. We speak good and bad people. Related to these terms may be mentally normal or abnormal terms. Well-coordinated people are considered successful in the art of life.

Amrania (2010) Compiled A Specific Definition of Adaptation

Adaptation is the result of personal efforts to deal with stress and meet needs. Personal adaptation is the process of interaction between us and our environment. This process allows you to adapt or change your situation. Satisfying personal coordination depends on the success of the dialogue—a state where unique and environmental needs to be fully there and harmony between individuals and goals.

Woleman

It is a harmonious relationship with the environment involving the ability to satisfy most of one's needs and meet the demands.

Areas of Adjustment

For an individual, adaptation consists of both personal and environmental factors. These two aspects of adjustment move into smaller elements of personal and environmental factors. Adaptations appear as universal characteristics or qualities but can have different features and aspects. Numerous efforts to measure customization through inventory and other techniques have identified these aspects and created various tests to assess their dimensions. For example, Bell (1958) recorded five dimensions in his adaptive inventory: home, health, social, emotional, and professional.

Arkoff (1968) cited family, school or college, profession, and marriage as essential areas of adaptation. A research study on students in Joshi and Pandey (1964). It was specified measuring range for adjustment of 11 people.

1. Health and physical development.

2. Finance, living conditions, and employment.

3. Social and leisure activities.

4. Advertising, sex, marriage.

5. Social and psychological relationships.

6. Personal psychological relationships.

7. Moral and religious.

8. Home and family.

9. Future-oriented and educational.

10. Adaptation to school and college work.

11. Curriculum and instruction.

Thus, Personal and environmental factors work in parallel to achieve this harmony.

Characteristics of A Well-Adjusted Person

A well-tuned person should have the following features:

1. Recognize your strengths and limitations: Well-tuned people know their strengths and weaknesses. In some areas, they seek to harness his assets by accepting his limits in other areas.

2. Respect for yourself and others: Dislike yourself is a typical symptom of disagreement. Adapted people respect themselves and others.

3. Enough suction level: The suction level is neither too low nor too high regarding the strengths and abilities.

Don't try to reach for the stars. Also, do not regret choosing the natural course for the ascent.

4. Satisfaction with basic needs: The basic organic, emotional, and social needs are either fully satisfied or a process of achievement. The person does not suffer from personal desires and social isolation. He feels relatively safe and maintains self-esteem.

5. Lack of critical or false attitude: He appreciates the goodness of objects, people, or activities. He does not seek weaknesses or mistakes. His observations are more specific than critical or punitive. He likes people, admires their goodness, and wins their love.

6. Behavioral flexibility: There is no rigorous evidence about the attitude or way of life. People can quickly adapt to changing circumstances by making the necessary changes to the actions.

7. Ability to deal with adversity: It is not easily overwhelmed by difficulty and has the willingness and courage to resist and fight adversity. The person has a fundamental urge to learn his environment rather than passively accepting it.

8. Realistic perception of the world: It has a natural vision and has no obligation to escape the imagination. The person always thinks systematically and acts practically.

9. Ambient brightness: Adaptable People are happy with their surroundings. It fits nicely in the home, family, neighborhood, and other social environments. When the person enters the profession, he loves it and retains his enthusiasm despite all adversity.

10. Balanced Philosophy of Life: A well-coordinated person has a philosophy that gives direction to life while at the same time, considering changing situations and situational requirements. This philosophy focuses on his environment, his culture, and his demands so that he does not conflict with himself.

Theory and Model of Adaptation

Why do some people adapt to their environment, and others do not? What are the factors that adjust or mismatch a person? Some various theories and models explain the adjustment patterns to answer such questions.

1. Moral model: This is the oldest perspective on adaptation or mismatch. In this view,

adjustments or inconsistencies should be there morally, that is, on the absolute norm of expected behavior. Those who follow the code are adjusted, and those who violate or do not follow these codes are wrongly changed (sinners). The evil supernatural powers of demons, etc. have been accused of violating norms (sinking). Still, religious gods, goddesses, and other holy and great souls make people happy to make people healthy, prosperous, and pious (adapted in a modern sense), however, as medical and biological sciences progress, scientific thinking.

In the 19th century, moral models got replaced by medical and natural models.

2. Medical-biological model: This model includes genetic, physiological, and biochemical factors that cause individuals who are or having low esteem with themselves and their environment. According

to this model, mismatches are the result of diseases of body tissues, especially the brain. Such conditions can be the result of inheritance or damage that has occurred in the course of a person's life-injuries, infections or disorders in which it is necessary to correct the defective tissue by physical therapy such as drugs, surgery.

This model is still extant and enjoys credibility for rooting out the causes of failure in terms of genetic influences, biochemical defect hypotheses, and disease in the tissues of the body. However, it is not correct to assign physiological or organic causes to all maladjusted and malfunctioning behavior, especially when there is no evidence of physiological malfunction. Such a situation indeed calls for other explanations, viewpoints, or models.

The Psychoanalytical Model

This model owes its origin to the theory of psychoanalysis propagated by Sigmund Freud and supported by psychologists like Adler, Jung, and other neo-Freudians.

Sigmund Freud's View

a) The human psyche or mind consists of three layers, the conscious, the subconscious, and the unconscious. The unconscious holds the key to our behavior. It decides the individual's adjustment and maladjustment to himself and his environment. It contains all the repressed wishes, desires, feelings, drives, and motives, many of which are related to sex and aggression. One is adjusted or maladjusted to the degree, extent, or how these are kept dormant or under control.

b) According to Freud, man is a pleasure-seeking animal by nature. He wants to seek pleasure and avoids pain or anything which is not in keeping with his fun-loving personality. The social restrictions imposed by the moral of society and his ethical standards dictated by his superego come in conflict with the unrestricted and unbridled desires of his essential pleasure-seeking nature. These pleasures are mostly sexual. One remains adjusted to the extent that these are satisfied. An individual drift towards malfunctioning of behavior and maladjustment in case such satisfaction is threatened or denied. Freud formulated the following conclusion:

A person's behavior remains normal and in harmony with his self and his environment to the extent that his ego can maintain the balance between the evil designs of his id and the oral ethical standard dictated by his superego. In case the ego is not strong enough to exercise proper control over one's id and superego, the malfunction of behavior would result. Two different situations could then arise.

I. If the superego dominates, then there is no acceptable outlet for the experience of the repressed wishes, impulses, and appetites of the id. Such a situation may give birth to neurotic tendencies in the individual.

I. If the id dominates, then the individual pursues his unbridled pleasure-seeking impulses, without care of the engaged in unlawful or immoral activities resulting in maladaptive, problem or delinquent behavior.

c) Freud also uses the concept of libido, i.e., a flow of energy-related to sexual gratification. He equates it with a flowing river and maintains that:

I. If its flow is outward, causing sex gratification and pleasurable sensation from external objects, the individual remains relatively healthy and adjusted to his self and the environment.

II. If it flows inward, then it leads to self-indulgence and narcissism.

III. If its path is blocked, this results in its arrest leading to regressive behavior, a kind of abnormality.

IV. If the flow of the libido turns out as dammed, condemned, or repressed through the authority exercised by the ego. The ego performs this function in association with the superego; it may cause severe maladjustment. When the ego is weak, and the superego is rigid, this may lead to psychotic personality disorders. However, when the ego is fragile, and the superego is also not too severe, it may result in relatively simple complications. The intricacies can be neurosis or still more specific maladaptive behavior. The behaviors characterized by restlessness, sleeplessness, headache, stomachache, backache, vomiting, lack of appetite, etc.

d) According to Freud, adjustment or maladjustment should not be viewed only in terms of what the individual may be undergoing at present. What happened to him in his earlier childhood is even more critical. What the person may have experienced as a child, and how he has passed through the distinct stages of Sexual development, etc., are quite famous for making him adjusted or maladjusted to his self and the environment.

Adler's Views

Adler disagreed with his teacher and replaced the original motif with a desire to achieve superiority and completeness to explain the motives of power or human behavior. He claimed that all people have a strong urge to seek an advantage for power. Besides, because they are helpless and dependent as a child, they feel a sense of inferiority and resort to compensatory behavior to compensate for the deficiency. In other words, let go of the power struggle. Environmental conditions, weak constitution, and many other factors can make you feel sick. To escape these feelings, you learn to fight for power. Individual efforts to seek power and achieve perfection require the need for creative expression, the urge to do something new, the desire to improve one's status in the eyes of peers and others. It also comes from passion.

b) In this way, envisioning an unmistakable lifestyle that responds to your environmental situation, inspired by the urge to pursue power or to achieve excellence and integrity. People continue to pursue excellence by imitating and utilizing the means and methods of their lifestyle. Adaptation or lack of adjustment depends on the success of your efforts to achieve your goals. Three situations can occur:

I. Successful pursuit of motives for gaining power and superiority leads to successful adaptation to oneself and the environment.

II. If a partial failure succeeds in making a small change in your life goals and lifestyle, you may be able to harmonize yourself with the environment, feel adjusted, and stay regular.

III. Unfulfilled power motives and changing goals and lifestyles can lead to inappropriate or inappropriate behavior leading to mild or severe mental illness.

Jung's View

Jung's system of analytical psychology supported Freud's quest for self-realization instead of the motive for sexual satisfaction and Adler's quest for power to explain human behavior. According to him, a person has a strong inner urge or motive to show his talents or skills or seek self-fulfillment. Therefore, to satisfy the impulse of self-actualization, one uses one's life energy, that is, the flow of libido as a pathway for self-expression. The degree of adaptation of your personality depends on how successful you are in achieving your personal. The vital energy that Jung maintains, libido can flow inward or outward, transforming an individual into an introverted or extroverted character.

But in general, individuals are not purely introverts or extroverts. It's all around. That is, they show introverted symptoms.

Extroversion has several characteristics and vice versa. If a person can maintain the right balance of thoughts and emotions, he will remain acclimatized to himself and his environment. However, one-sided behavior— too much emphasis on theories at the expense of feelings, or excessive consideration of compassion at the expense of thoughts can upset your mental balance. It can lead to mismatches leading to mild or severe mental illness.

Another criterion of normal or adequately adaptable behavior, according to Jung's theory, is reconciliation between conscious and unconscious behavior. If someone fails to maintain or achieve such an agreement, it can lead to discord and mental illness. When consciousness is not in harmony with unconsciousness, or when unconsciousness becomes hostile because it is not adequately understandable employing the of knowledge, it creates an imbalance in mind. It makes behavior towards itself and its environment very evil. When this hostility or aggression turns inward, it becomes neurotic, and when it overflows, it causes psychosis and delinquency. As Jung argues, in some forms of dangerous madness, complete unconscious autonomy, a sort of total control, or a conscious bombing of unconscious content with disturbing content is found.

Karen Horny View

Adler believed that the need for power (to counter inferiority) was the leading cause of human behavior, but Horny (1937) needed safety (to offset the feeling of fear). As a child, she assumed that individuals felt helpless and isolated in a potentially hostile world. It creates some underlying fear and his need for security. Ethical security issues are typical. However, when an individual is safely possessed and interferes with self-development, she tends to behave inconsistently or abnormally.

Anxious children can continue to doubt and eventually move towards and depend on a person, push against them, become hostile and rebellious, or pull themselves away from others. If a person can incorporate these three attitudes or answers, sometimes give, sometimes fight, sometimes if he stays for himself, he can continue to adapt himself and his surroundings. However, looking at one of these directions, regardless of their suitability in a situation, can lead to poor adaptation and mild or severe mental illness or criminal conduct.

According to Horney's theory, there is a reason for disagreement. That is the rejection or obstruction of the pathway. He said that there is a conflict between your ideal self and your true self. Individuals can remain tuned and healthy enough to maintain the right balance between these two selves and, if disturbed, may drift to abnormal or poorly coordinated movements.

Erich Fromm View

Like Horny, Fromm emphasizes the need for safety and believes that as a child, you can feel the need to belong to balance the fear of isolation and loneliness. But when he was mature, he was driven by an inner desire for freedom, thus trying to escape the bond that gave him the necessary security? In such a situation, he may face an internal conflict of reliance on meeting his need for safety and his need for freedom.

Members also go through certain situations that give their offspring independence to play a mature role and try to retain them to ensure future security. The extent to which this crisis of freedom from children or dependence on safety finds a solution with the help of parents and elders determines how well their behavior and function are regulated and remain rational. If this crisis is not fully steadfast, there will be disagreements followed by mental illness and criminal character formation.

Wilhelm Reich View

Consistent with Freud's view of sexual importance, Reich declared firmly that the physical and mental health of an individual depended on the release of a sexual drive to orgasm. However, from the day of birth, the escape of libido and sexual energy from parents, teachers, and society, in general, is thwarted. Reich considered the term "sexual energy" in a broader sense and called it "Orgon energy." It is the vital force that stimulates an individual's overall behavior and is responsible for all kinds of self-expression. When this energy is directed correctly and flows in the standard, the individual remains healthy and enjoys good physical and mental health. However, blocking the flow of energy can cause physical discomfort first, followed by physiological and psychological disability, which can lead to mild to severe disagreement and mental illness.

Ericsson VIEW

Ericsson views adaptation as a function of the conflict between innate instincts and social demands. He divided the entire human life into eight different stages. In each phase, societies formed by specific cultures make specific demands. It addresses the instinct that an individual reveals during this phase. In this way, at every stage of life, a crisis can be faced, and its solution can have a positive or negative effect on adaptation. For example, as a child, individuals face the problem of resolving the crisis inherent in that stage. That is trust (which allows us to build intimate relationships) and distrust (which will enable us to protect ourselves in a hostile world). Its proper growth and development. The consequences of the actions depend on the success or failure of a satisfactory solution to this crisis, which may result in developing into a healthy personality or an incomplete and deviant character.

Social or Cultural Model

According to this model, societies in general and culture have a strong influence on their behavior, so behavior takes the form of adaptive or non-adaptive behavior that transforms you into an adaptive or non-adaptive personality. The society and culture in which you belong not only influence and shape your practice but also set the criteria for how your followers behave in the way you want. Individuals that act as society wants 50 deviations from social norms, and violations of role expectations are considered signs of mismatches or abnormalities but ascribe to as usual and adapted individuals. Society and culture play essential roles in shaping and influencing human behavior, but this should not be the only factor in the mismatch process. Moreover, the communities and cultures themselves, not the individual, are not able to adapt well, even destroying the adaptations of individuals. Therefore, it is not appropriate to rely solely on social or cultural models to mark one's behavior as adapted or under-adapted.

Social psychology or behavioral models generally emphasize this.

I. Behavior is not inherited. The abilities needed to succeed in life are acquired or learned by the individual, primarily through social experience.

II. While the environmental impact of cultural and social institutions is essential, it is their interaction with the physical and social environment or their psychological self that plays a crucial role in determining the success or failure of adaptation.

III. Behaviors, whether regular or abnormal, are learned according to the same learning principles or rules. In general, each type of behavior is discovered or acquired as resulting aftermath. You can learn to consider answers marked as usual as abnormal.

IV. Not only is normal and abnormal behavior learned, but it also labels behavior as routine as strange. If a person examines, an unusual tuned to action depends on the observer's practice and social context of the behavior.

V. Inconsistent behavior can hold forth by the application of principles or behavioral changes, lack of learning, deterioration of conditions, and modification of the environmental conditions that cause them.

All the above models are correct, except for some primordial moral models to explain the success or failure of adjustments. But none of them is enough to provide a satisfactory explanation of whether it is completed. Medical or biological models offer a reasonable basis for understanding mental illness or inconsistent behavior caused by organic causes, physical brain damage, and genetic factors, but psychological causes and social. It cannot solicit into failure due to factors. Adaptation must always be a continuous product of the interaction of biological and genetic structures with the natural and social determinants of the environment. Therefore, it is innate and learned. For analysis, the analysts must investigate an individual's interactions with the current climate, his past, his conflicts, and crises. Therefore, you can comprehensively view the above models to explain and understand them.

Adjustment Method

To live a healthy, happy, and satisfying life, we need to learn different types of adaptation. To understand these methods, we need to consider the possible modes, techniques, and practices that individuals may use in the adaptation process.

There are two categories, direct and indirect:

Direct Method

The direct method is a method that is intentionally used by an individual at a conscious level. They are rational and logical and help to solve the problems individuals face in certain situations permanently. The methods include:

(A) Trial Error and Improved Effort: If you find it difficult to solve a problem or encounter a disability along the way, you can reinforce your efforts and improve your behavioral process with new enthusiasm.

(B) Compromise: You can make the following compromises to keep yourself in harmony with the environment.

1) You can change direction entirely by replacing the original goal. That is, a public servant aspirant of the country can turn the

power to become a probation officer for a state-owned bank.

2) Instead of Indian administrative services, you can request a partial exchange of destinations, such as the choice of local civil servants.

3) You can be satisfied with the obvious alternative to the real thing. For children, arms instead of a real car, if the boy wants to marry the doll.

(C) Withdrawal and Obedience: You can learn how to deal with the environment by accepting the defeat and yielding to the powerful forces of the environment and the situation.

(D) Make Appropriate Decisions: A person adapts to his surroundings, using his intelligence to make appropriate and wise decisions, especially in conflict, stressful situations, and Seeking harmony.

Indirect Method

The indirect method is a temporary attempt to adapt to protect yourself from psychological dangers. These are purely subjective or spiritual. A way of perceiving the situation he wants to see and imagining it to happen. Therefore, they are called defensive or mental mechanisms used in the process of adapting to yourself and the environment. Some essential psychological tools are:

a) Repression: Repression is a mechanism by which painful experiences, conflicts, and unfulfilled desires shove into the unconsciousness. In this way, you unknowingly try to forget what might make him anxious or offensive. Believing that there is no tension-creating situation, they try to relieve tension and fear temporarily.

b) Regression: Regression means going back in the past. In this process, individuals tend to rely on early childhood or early childhood reactions to protect themselves from mental conflicts and tensions. A man who fails a romantic relationship retreats when he shows his love for the doll. Similarly, older children can retract and behave like infants when they feel their new siblings were born and ignored.

c) Compensation: This is a mechanism that seeks to make up for or hide a shortage in one area by showing strength in another city. For example, an unattractive girl who becomes a bookworm and secures her position in the class uses such a mechanism to attract attention that her appearance cannot.

d) Rationalization: This is a defensive mechanism that justifies behavior by giving a person a reason for social acceptance, and thus a plausible excuse to explain their behavior. People try to protect themselves by doing. Children use rationalization when trying to extend an incomplete explanation due to failure.

Children can blame the teacher, parents, or his illness to hide his weaknesses and deficiencies.

e) Projection: Through projection, we attempt to see or attribute our inferior urges or characteristics of other people or objects. Clumsy people see and criticize other people's awkwardness. Similarly, students who have gone through the process of testing can be confident that others have committed fraud. A person with a strong unsatisfactory sexual drive may blame others for sexual goals or try to think in the world around them. In this way, you try to overlook or defend your shortcomings by emphasizing what others are worse than him.

f) Identity: If you use this mechanism as an individual, you will be satisfied with its success by verifying your identity with other people, groups, or institutions. Artists who have yet to succeed in his field can eke out with established artists. You can match your school and be proud of its fame and reputation. Similarly, hero worship is another form of personal identification with famous leaders and film actors. He imitates his characteristics, clothes, and manners and enjoys his achievements and success.

g) Isolation or withdrawal: Using this mechanism, one tends to withdraw from a situation that causes frustration or failure. He is safe and secure by running away from the problem. For example, because of fear of failure, a child can refuse to participate in the game and, if they do, believe in success and cheat themselves. Fantasy is a kind of fiction and makes you feel.

Instead of being threatened by reality, you can be content with unrealistic fictitious success in the world of appearance and imagination.

h) Empathy: Empathy is a defense mechanism in which an individual seeks satisfaction by seeking compassion for their mistakes and shortcomings. Such people are continually increasing difficulties and obstacles on their way to success and persuading others to feel sorry for them. For example, a housewife who doesn't raise a child well stimulates the compassion of others by telling her family isn't working with her or how the family is struggling and how she overworked.

All the above defense mechanisms are used by one person unknowingly (even if for the time being) to protect themselves from psychological danger. They are not a permanent cure for the problem. As Morgan says, "They hide the real problem. It's still there. Ready to create fear many times" (Amraniya, 2010). Therefore, the defense mechanism can contemplate as a temporary defense against anxiety and deficiency.

Moreover, the use of such a device may introduce new difficulties for those who use it. It's like telling a lie to protect yourself from a difficult situation and take a break, but it's uncomfortable because of a false statement. It should monitor closely. Children understand that they do not use such defense mechanisms frequently.

CONCLUSION

Psychic Empath is not just about a lack of mental illness. It is a complete and harmonious function of the whole personality. People in emotional, physical, and social well-being fulfill their responsibilities in their lives, role virtually in their daily lives, and are content with interpersonal relationships.

A sane child feels good about himself, enjoys his relationships, learns with confidence, and overcomes his difficulties. Some children are overwhelmed by misery, anger, or fear. According to a study, up to 10% of children in the 5 to the 15-year-old group have mental disorders. In most cases, these are the companions with considerable stress and considerable impairment of individual functioning. Children with mental health problems usually cannot even learn effectively.

Between the ages of 12 and 18, changes in body shape, development of secondary sexual characteristics, hormonal and biochemical alterations form the basis of mature sexual function. Due to the changes, they are experiencing, adolescents are beginning to revise their views on themselves. Social relationships outside the family are becoming increasingly important. It is not uncommon to rebel against the authority of parents during adolescence. Strange but true, youth is the most challenging generation for adolescents to find their identity easily.

All of this involves continuous change and adaptation to your environment. Adaptation consists of both personal and environmental elements. These two aspects of adjustment can split into smaller parts of personal and environmental factors. Transformation appears to be a universal characteristic or characteristic, but it can have different dimensions. These aspects figure out the various tests intend to evaluate their dimensions.

Almost all a child's experience during the first few years is usually related to home and school. These two institutions are more responsible for children's mental health and educational coordination than any other. Therefore, it is essential to consider the mental health and academic adjustment of children in this age group. Numerous studies of mental health, adaptation, and related concepts disseminate at international, national, and state levels.

COPYRIGHTS

This book

"Psychic Empath: Psychic Development Survival Guide for Highly Sensitive People. Practicing Mindfulness, Mental Health Essential Meditations and Affirmations to Reduce Stress and Find Your Sense of Self

Written by Jack Gross

This document is intended to provide accurate and authoritative details about the subject and the issue under discussion. This product is sold on the assumption that no officially approved bookkeeping or publishing company offers any other available resources. If you need a legal or qualified guide, that person must have the right to join the field. A policy statement, a subcommittee of the American Bar Association, a committee of publishers and associations, is approved. No part of this text may be reproduced, duplicated, or distributed electronically or in writing.

The recording of this document is strictly prohibited. This text can be retained only with the written approval of the publisher and all free approval. The information provided herein is intended to reflect the lack of attention or other means resulting from the misuse or use of the procedures, procedures, or instructions contained therein, and the general and absolute obligations of the target user. Accurate and reliable.

The author has no direct or indirect liability or liabilities for recovery, damage, or loss resulting from the data collected here. Each author reserves all copyright not owned by the publisher. The information contained herein is generally available for informational purposes only. The data are presented without any guarantee or promise of any kind. The trademarks used are used without permission and are patented without the consent or protection of the patentee. The logos and labels in this book are the property of their owners and are not linked to this text.

CPSIA information can be obtained
at www.ICGtesting.com
Printed in the USA
BVHW061053170621
609821BV00002B/182

9 781802 765137